Avascular Necrosis (Osteonecrosis)

The Silent, Rare Disease:

My Story

by Wyketha K Parkman

DEDICATION

I dedicate this book to all of my family, friends and to all that are going through the stages of this silent rare disease Avascular Necrosis.

CONTENTS

Acknowledgments i

1   Chapter 1   Pg #1

2   Chapter 2   Pg #6

3   Chapter 3   Pg #10

4   Chapter 4   Pg #16

5   Chapter 5   Pg #22

6   Chapter 6   Pg #27

7   Chapter 7   Pg #33

8   Chapter 8   Pg #38

9   Chapter 9   Pg #44

10 Chapter 10   Pg #53

11 Chapter 11   Pg #64

12 Chapter 12   Pg #71

13 Chapter 13   Pg #78

14 Chapter 14   Pg #87

15 Chapter 15   Pg #98

16 Chapter 16   Pg #109

Diagnostic Tests   Pg #119

Epilogue   Pg #122

Images   Pg #124

About the author   Pg #136

Reference   Pg #133

ACKNOWLEDGMENTS

I started a petition to acknowledge Avascular Necrosis for it's disabling state. Please help me to get this approve by the White House by going to the link below. All is needed is your first and last name, email address and zip code. You can share the petition via email and text. Let's makes this happen.

Thank you in advance.

https://sign.moveon.org/petitions/awareness-for-the-disease

Chapter 1

In 2014, I was diagnosed with avascular necrosis of the hips. That's when my nightmare began.

What is avascular necrosis?

Avascular necrosis (AVN), also known as osteonecrosis of the femoral head, occurs when the blood supply to the bone is decreased. This interruption in blood supply causes small cracks and breaks in the bone. If the AVN is left untreated, the bone will eventually die and collapse.

Over 20,000 people acquire AVN every year, typically between 20 and 50 years old. It can be caused by a number of factors, such as damage to the bone's blood supply, or injury to the bone itself, which can damage blood vessels and precipitate AVN. Other potential causes include prolonged and frequent use of corticosteroids, hip dislocation or fracture, inflammation, blood clots, sickle cell anemia, pancreatitis, HIV, excessive alcohol intake, chemotherapy/radiation therapy, and leukemia. Healthy people have a smaller risk of developing AVN.

AVN commonly occurs in the hips, but can also develop in the knees, ankles, and shoulders. The symptoms of AVN include hip pain, especially when the hip is bearing excessive weight, and pain in the groin, buttocks, and down the front of the thigh. The pain eventually intensifies, causing limping, joint stiffness, inflammation, and restlessness when trying to sleep.

My story

On March 05, 2005, I was admitted into one of the hospitals in Houston, Texas, with severe pain in my lower back and in both legs. I can remember it like it was yesterday.

A few hours after I had an MRI scan of my head, with and without contrast (a test that generates detailed images of the brain, using magnetic fields and radio waves), I started experiencing severe pain in my lower back and in both upper legs. At home, I tried soaking in the bathtub filled with hot water, Epsom salt and rubbing alcohol. Since that had always been an effective home remedy for sore, swollen, painful, aching bones and joints, I thought I should give it a try. That didn't ease the pain, so I took two Aleves, since it was also known to help with painful, sore, aching bones and joints. That didn't help either. I was in so much pain, I could barely walk.

I tried to figure out what I had done to cause so much pain, but the only thing I could think of was being diagnosed with a sinus infection and a high fever. I slowly walked over to my bed and eased myself down to sit. I must have sat there for over 30 minutes before I had the courage to lie down. The pain was so intense and severe in my lower back that I cried. I finally got the courage to lie down. I grabbed onto my headboard and pulled myself as close to it as I could manage. I then grabbed onto my right leg, lifting it until I got it in the bed. Next, I grabbed hold of my left leg and did the same thing. I sat up in my bed with my back against the wall and headboard for several minutes, trying to ignore the excruciating pain by watching television. I looked over at my husband who was sleeping so peacefully and wished I could do the same.

I began to notice that I was rocking myself, trying to ease the pain. I rocked back and forth, trying desperately to get some kind of relief, but it didn't help. I tried waking my husband by pushing on him, but my touch was too weak and soft. I thought to myself, I need to go to the Emergency Room because something was not right. Why would I be experiencing all of this pain when I hadn't done anything to cause it? I didn't fall, and I wasn't injured. It had to be something that was causing this horrible pain. I prayed to God it wasn't something serious or fatal.

I walked over to my closet, grabbed a pair of pants, a bra, a shirt, and my shoes. As I was getting dressed, the tears flowed down my face from all of the pain. I just kept praying, God, whatever I have done for you to cause me so much pain, please spare me and forgive me for it.

After I was dressed, I grabbed my purse, jacket and keys. I looked back at my husband who was still sleeping so peacefully in the bed, and walked out of our bedroom. I went into my two sons' room and they were also asleep. I stood in their door for about five minutes, and then walked out.

Once I got to the front door, I dreaded going out the door. You see, at the time, we lived in a three-bedroom apartment that was on the second floor. I walked out the door, closed it behind me, and locked it. When I looked down at my car, the tears flowed faster down my face. I had to walk down two flights of stairs. All I could do was ask for the strength and balance to get me down every step without falling, because I didn't need an injury in addition to not knowing what was causing all of this pain. I cried and moaned all the way down the stairs until I got to the bottom. I unlocked the car door with the keyless entry remote, threw my purse and jacket on the passenger side, and sat in the driver's seat. I grabbed my right leg and swung it into the car. The pain was so intense and excruciating, I screamed out, dreading putting the other leg in. But I had no choice in the matter if I wanted to get to the Emergency Room to see what was wrong with me and find out what was causing all of this pain. I took in several breaths, grabbed my left leg, and swung it into the car. I just wanted someone to knock me out because I was in so much pain.

I closed the door, started the car, turned on the heater, and sat for a minute or two so the engine could warm up. After for a few minutes, I put the car in reverse and slightly pressed on the gas pedal, but, oh, the pain! I screamed so loud, I thought I woke up some of my neighbors. The pain radiated from my lower back, down the side of my right leg to the top of my knees. I pressed on the brake, put the car in drive, and slightly pressed the gas pedal. The pain was excruciating. I just kept screaming out, "God, if you can, please hear my cry! I am in so much pain, God! I don't know how much more I can tolerate. If you can, please just ease the pain until I can get to the hospital!"

Houston has so many hospitals, but I drove to the one closest to my apartment. I drove 75 mph going to the hospital. I was so happy there was no traffic. The best time to travel in Houston is early morning, hours before the sun comes up.

It was around 1:23 am when I started to make my way to the hospital. Within ten minutes, I was pulling into the Emergency Room's patient parking lot. I was able to park close to the door. I dreaded pressing the brakes, but I knew I had to if I wanted to stop the car and turn it off. I slightly pushed the brakes and put the car in park. I turned off the heater, grabbed my purse and jacket, opened the door, and grabbed my left leg, swinging it out of the car. I then grabbed my right leg and swung it out. The pain, that excruciating pain! It felt like someone was drilling into my lower back, leg bones, and joints, and I cried out. After a moment, I braced myself with both of my hands and lifted my body out of the car, then closed the door and pressed the car alarm to lock it.

I took a few tiny steps, but for some reason, my legs were not following my brain's orders.

(If you're familiar with anatomy, you may know that motor functions are controlled mainly by the primary motor cortex via neural impulses.)

I stopped and stood in one spot with tears running freely down my face because of the pain. It took all the strength and energy I had to take another step. I thought to myself, I can't let my mental state take control because if it did, I wasn't going to take another step.

When I wiped my eyes, I noticed a medical employee looking at me. I just stood there, not able to get my legs and feet to cooperate with me. I screamed out, "Move! Please move!"

I heard a male voice say, "Ma'am, I am here to help you. I have a wheelchair. Can you please sit in it for me?"

I stopped crying and tried to do what he asked. As I got ready to sit in the wheelchair, the pain got at least five times worse. I couldn't move any further, I couldn't sit in the wheelchair. Then I heard another voice, this time a female.

"Ma'am, I can see you are in severe pain, but I need you to have a seat so we can get you in to see the doctor. Where does it hurt?"

I told her, crying, "My lower back and both of my legs."

"Okay, just take your time sitting in the wheelchair, you are almost there," she said. Finally, after what seemed like forever, I sat in the wheelchair. That was a huge mistake. I screamed out in agony! The woman kept saying she was sorry. She told me they were going to get me some kind of relief.

Once we were inside the hospital, the man rolled me into an exam room. I can vaguely remember being asked for my personal information, if I had medical insurance, or even an emergency contact.

Then another male voice was saying, "I am a doctor. From 1 to 10, what is your pain level?"

I answered, "I had two natural births without epidurals and I'd rather be having contractions instead of this pain!"

The doctor asked, "Are you allergic to anything I should be aware of?"

I told him, "Doxycycline."

He immediately asked the nurse to arrange a room for me upstairs, stat, an IV (intravenous, within vein) and morphine. He explained to me that he was admitting me for further testing and was going to start an IV to start giving me morphine for the pain. The nurse walked back in, set me up with the IV, and pushed the morphine through the tube. The last question I remember the doctor asking me was for a phone number to reach my husband. I don't remember anything after that.

Chapter 2

I remember waking up to voices around me. I slowly opened my eyes and the first person I saw was my husband. He was talking to a nurse. He came over and kissed me on my forehead, asking me how I was doing.

"How are you feeling today?" asked the nurse.

"Oh, I don't know," I answered. "Well, I feel like I've been hit by a bus."

"It's the pain medication, the morphine," the nurse explained.

I was surprised. "The morphine! I get sick to the stomach if I take hydrocodone, yet I was given morphine? How can that be?"

"It was your pain level," said the nurse. "It states in your chart that upon admission, your pain level was comparable to contractions when giving birth. Do you recall any of this? Do you remember anything prior to waking up?"

"Yes, I do. I remember that horrible, excruciating pain in my lower back and both of my legs. I also remember trying to get some relief at home by soaking in my bathtub filled with hot water, Epsom salt, and green rubbing alcohol. I also remember trying to wake him up," I pointed to my husband, "because of the pain. I remember getting dressed, walking down those stairs, getting into the car, driving here, being pushed in a wheelchair by a woman and a man who met me in the parking lot by my car because the pain kept me from walking."

"Do you remember anything else prior to talking to the admitting physician?"

"Yes, I remember him asking about my pain level, my husband's phone number, and if I was allergic to anything."

The nurse smiled. "You have a great memory. Well, there's nothing wrong with that."

"What day is today?" I asked. "How long have I been here?"

"Today is Sunday. You came in the early morning."

"Has the doctor found out what was causing the pain?"

"No, you are scheduled to have several tests," said the nurse. "We have also collected blood to make sure all of your levels are normal and to make sure you don't have any other type of illness."

"This is so strange. Why would I be experiencing this type of pain? Unless...?" I paused.

"Unless, what?"

"I have a half-sister on my father's side who just told me several weeks ago she was diagnosed with lupus," I explained. (Lupus is a chronic, autoimmune disease in which the body's immune system attacks its own healthy cells and tissues, resulting in inflammation and pain.) "Could that be it? I do know with that disease, it can be years before being diagnosed; you have to be experiencing the symptoms to be tested and it is hereditary."

"I will let the doctor know," the nurse assured me. "Someone will be in here shortly to give you your medications. Are you experiencing any pain now? What is your pain level from 1 – 10?"

"It is 6."

She checked her watch. "It's time for a dose of your morphine. I will make sure they give you that, too."

I thanked the nurse, and she left the room.

My husband came to sit on the side of my bed. "How are you feeling?" he asked.

"I am better than I was last night, or whenever it was," I answered.

"Why didn't you wake me up?"

"I tried," I told him. "But you were knocked out from having a few drinks with my cousin while watching the game."

He took my hand. "I am sorry. I didn't know. I made sure you were alright after coming home from your MRI with your mother."

"I know and it is alright." I squeezed his hand. "I lived through it all. No harm was done except for that pain."

For seven days, I was in the hospital having every test you could think of on my lower back and both legs. I had MRIs with and without contrast, X-rays, CT scans, lab work and Dopplers. In addition to all of these tests, I was tested for lupus and sickle cell anemia. But they couldn't find the cause or make a diagnosis.

The Thursday before I was discharged, one of the nurses came in to give me my medications. I knew by the color of one of the pills that it was to treat depression. My current job at the time was a medical assistant with the job description of a nurse. I asked her how long I'd been taking that medication. I had never looked at my medications until that particular moment. She started stuttering when she tried to answer me. I explained to her that I was in my right state of mind and I had the right to know when they had started giving me that medication and why I was taking it. She finally admitted it was given to me for depression. I immediately explained to her that couldn't be true because the doctors couldn't find out what was causing the pain. I asked her to please let the doctor know I was refusing to take the medication for depression.

I was discharged from the hospital without a diagnosis, but I had a prescription for Vicodin to be taken as directed for the pain, and discharge papers to follow up with my primary care doctor. For several days, I was able to manage the pain I was experiencing. For once, I was able to tolerate it.

When I returned to work, the doctor I worked for performed an EMG (electromyography) on both of my legs. (An EMG is a diagnostic test used to evaluate how your muscles and motor neurons (the nerve cells that control the muscles) are functioning. The electrical activity of the motor neurons is recorded and analyzed to determine whether the patient has a muscle or nerve disorder, such as sciatica, sclerosis, or muscular dystrophy.) The test didn't show anything abnormal. The results were normal.

Days, weeks, months and years went by without experiencing any pain like I had experienced in the year 2005. I was no longer taking the Vicodin for pain. Every now and then, the doctors I worked for (neurologists who specialize in disorders affecting the brain, spinal cord, and nerves) asked me how I was doing. They would also ask if I had experienced any more pain like I did before. I would always tell them no. I would always say that the pain disappeared into thin air.

Chapter 3

In early June of 2013, we had family visiting us from out of town. For that week, I was off from work. Every day, we were doing something different. We played video games, some of which required physical movements: bowling, dancing, basketball and golf. A few days later, I started experiencing lower back pain and leg pain like I did back in 2005. I explained to my family what was going on with me. From there I started limiting my daily activities. Every day the pain started getting worse.

On July 4, 2013, the pain was severe in my lower back. I was lying in my bed when an excruciating, sharp pain moved from my lower back to the front of my hip, and down my right leg. The pain stopped at the end of my knee. It did not go any further. I told my husband that if it got worse, I was going to the Emergency Room (ER) in the morning. During the beginning of the night, I couldn't get to sleep. I had already taken two Aleves and a hot bath with Epsom salt and alcohol. As I was trying to get out of the bathtub, the pain got even worse. I had to lift my body up out of the water and out of the bathtub. I got dressed and got back in the bed. The pain did not allow me to sleep that night. I was up the entire night.

Once morning came on July 5, 2013, right before the sun came up, I told my husband I needed to go to the ER. I explained to him that the pain I was experiencing was like the pain I had in 2005 when I was admitted into the hospital. The pain extended from my lower back around to my inner thigh, and down to my knees. For some reason, it never went past my knees. I just couldn't figure out why, and neither could the doctors. After I spoke to my husband, I went into the bathroom, took a shower, got dressed, brushed my teeth, and brushed my hair. I grabbed my purse and told my husband I was ready to go.

Once we got to the hospital, it was a long wait before I saw the ER nurse. My husband and I were moved to two different areas in the ER before I was seen by a nurse. After an hour of sitting in that uncomfortable chair, I was finally called in.

The nurse asked to see the band they put around my wrist. "May I ask the reason why you are here this morning? What is your chief complaint?" she enquired.

"I am experiencing excruciating lower back pain and pain in both of my legs," I answered.

The nurse took down some notes. "Is this something new? Have you ever had pain in those areas before?"

"Yes, in 2005."

"What was the diagnosis?" she asked.

"They couldn't find out the reason for the pain," I told her. "No diagnosis was detected."

"From 1 – 10, what is your pain level right now?"

"More than 10," I answered.

"Would you like something for the pain? If so, have you eaten anything before you came in?"

"Yes, please, can you give me something for the pain? And yes, I had an apple."

"If you could please have a seat in the waiting area, and I will call you once I get the okay from the ER doctor to give you something for the pain."

I stood up slowly. "Okay, and thank you."

It seemed like I had been waiting forever when the nurse finally called me. She gave me a Vicodin for the pain and a small cup of water. She explained to me that someone was on their way to get me for some scans. She said that before she could do the X-ray, I had to take a pregnancy test to make sure I wasn't pregnant. I went into the bathroom, urinated in the cup, and took it back to her. She asked me to have a seat in the waiting area.

About an hour or so later, a porter came to escort me to do the scans. My husband followed. It seemed like it was taking forever to get to the designated area. I wanted to sit down so badly because I was in so much pain. We had to sit in another waiting area before I was called for the scans. But before the porter left, he wanted to make sure I was comfortable.

"Would you like a wheelchair?" he asked.

My husband answered for me, "Yes, if you don't mind."

The porter left the waiting area and within minutes, he returned with a wheelchair. He helped me sit down in it, then asked "Are you comfortable?"

I smiled gratefully. "I don't hurt as much, thank you."

There were four other people in the waiting area besides my husband and me, waiting to be called for their test. I started getting very uncomfortable sitting in the wheelchair. I started twisting, and turning, twisting and turning. I held back the tears from falling down my face. I wanted to cry and scream, but didn't. I just thought to myself, *If only I could cry and scream, maybe the noise would tune out the pain and I could ignore it.*

My husband was watching me, his brow furrowed with concern. "Baby, are you alright?"

"No!" I answered him, short and quick. The pain was wearing down my patience.

"Do you want me to go talk to someone so you can lie down?" my husband asked. "You look like you are in more pain sitting in that wheelchair."

I sighed in resignation. "I am, but I will be okay."

"No, it's not okay. We have been sitting here for an hour. Nobody has come in here to call anyone. What could be taking them so long?"

A lady sitting across from us said, "I have been sitting in here going on two hours. I think they have forgotten about us."

My husband stood up. "I will be back. I am going to see what's going on. They could at least have put you in a room where you could lie down until they come get you for the test."

He left the room, and within minutes, he was back with a nurse.

"Hello," she said. "I came to get you for your tests."

I just looked up at her. I didn't speak because I was in so much pain.

"How are you feeling now?" my husband asked.

"The pain feels as if it is getting worse," I gasped.

The nurse said, "I am going to unlock the wheelchair and push you to the testing room. I am sorry it took me so long to come and get you. There are so many people getting scans. We have several that came in by ambulance who had to get their scans first."

"I don't care about the ones that came in by ambulance," my husband retorted. "My wife has been here in pain since 7 am and it is after 12. I couldn't care less about the other people that are here. If she was here before them, she should have been first. If it wasn't an emergency, then we wouldn't be here. She should have been seen, given a diagnosis and medication, and sent on her way home by now."

"I do apologize, but I don't make the rules," the nurse said as she started wheeling me out of the waiting room.

Once we got to the testing room, another lady met me at the door. She asked if I could go in a room and remove my clothes and then cover up with a gown. I did what she asked. The pain was still severe even after taking the Vicodin. It hadn't eased the pain, not even a little. It seemed as if it was still getting worse. After I put the gown on, I went back into the room where the girl was. She gave me instructions on what to do for the scans she wanted. It was painful, but I survived. Once she was done, she checked the images to make sure she didn't have to repeat any of them. She asked me to get dressed and when I was done, she wheeled me back to where my husband was.

Once we got back to him, she had him follow us back to the waiting area where the nurse that gave me the Vicodin was. We sat there for another 30 minutes to an hour before I was called to a room. Once we were in the room, I tried lying down. Big mistake! That pain! It felt like someone was ripping me apart. The nurse asked if I wanted to take something for the pain. She looked at my chart and realized I had a Vicodin earlier in the day. She left the room and came back with another Vicodin and a small cup of water. I took the medicine and drank all of the water. She told me to try and lie down. She said the medication should kick in soon to help relieve the pain. She took another look at me, told me the doctor would be in shortly because I was next, and left.

Finally, the doctor came in with the results of my scans. "What do you think may be causing all of the pain?" he asked.

"I did some research and I think it's the sciatic nerve that's causing all of the pain," I answered.

The doctor flipped through the scan results. "That is what the scans shows, a pinched sciatic nerve."

"What can I do to stop all this pain? Can it be corrected? Will I need surgery?"

"I am going to give you two prescriptions," the doctor said. "One is for pain and one is a muscle relaxer until you can see your primary care doctor. The medications will help and surgery is not required."

"Can I return to work?" I asked.

The doctor nodded. "Yes, but light duty only, until you see your doctor."

"Can I have something in writing to give my boss, the doctor I work for?"

"Yes. I'll have the nurse bring it to you."

The doctor left the room. Within minutes, the nurse returned with my prescriptions and a note for work.

(The sciatic nerve, the largest nerve in the human body, runs from the lower back through the buttock and down the lower limb to the foot. It provides the vital connection from the leg, foot, and rear thigh muscles to the nervous system, via the spinal cord. Sciatica occurs when the sciatic nerve is irritated or compressed in the lower back. This can be caused by disc herniation, degenerative disc disease, or lumbar spinal stenosis, among other lower back and hip conditions. Symptoms of sciatica include pain radiating into the back of the thigh and calf, and extending down to the foot, as well as numbness, tingling, and burning sensations.)

My husband and I left the hospital feeling relieved. We finally knew what was causing the severe pain. Once I got in the car, I called and made an appointment to see my primary care doctor. When we got home, I took a shower because to sit in the tub was very painful. Once I was done, I got in my bed and curled up into a ball.

Chapter 4

The days and nights that went by before I saw my primary doctor were agonizing. The medications I was taking did not ease the pain. In fact, the pain only got worse. I wasn't getting any relief. The pain kept me from sleeping, and I didn't want to eat. It was painful to walk, sit up, and stand. I tried using ice packs, a heating pad, ointment for sore muscles and aching joints. I was taking Aleves, over-the-counter anti-inflammatory medications, pm medications to try to get some sleep. Everything I tried didn't help. I just didn't know what to do anymore. I was normally an energetic person. I had enough energy for two people. But with that pain, it slowed me completely down.

Two weeks after going to the ER, I was finally seeing my primary care doctor. As soon as I checked in, the nurse called me back to get my vitals. My husband followed us. (Vitals are the measurements of blood pressure, pulse, temperature, height and weight.) My blood pressure was elevated. It was 160/107 and my temperature was also high, 102.3. The nurse finished her assessment and took me to the exam room to wait for the doctor.

The doctor greeted me as she entered the exam room. She checked my chart and said, "I see you are here following up after your visit to the ER."

"Yes," I answered.

She looked back at the chart. "Let me see what they did over there and see what your diagnosis is."

"I was there for severe lower back pain which traveled around to the front of my legs down to my knees."

"I see here it's showing you are having problems with your sciatica."

"Yes, that's what they are saying."

"I want to get some blood to check your blood levels, and a urine test," the doctor said. "It is also showing your blood pressure is really high."

"I am sure it is because of the pain," I told her. "I never had high blood pressure before. My blood pressure is usually 110/59 or 119/59. It has always been on the low side. Some of the other doctors would make jokes as if I was walking dead. It has never been high. I know it's the pain."

"I want to put you on blood pressure medication temporarily until we can get it under control. I am not going to change the medication for the pain until after I get the results back on the lab work and urine."

I shook my head. "I don't want to be on blood pressure medication because I know it is elevated due to the pain."

"Just until you come back to follow up after your lab and urine results."

"Okay, if you say so. You are the doctor."

The doctor smiled. "Thank you. It's to keep you safe from a stroke or even a heart attack."

After the doctor examined me, my husband and I walked out of the exam room to the check-out desk. There, I was given my follow-up appointment. The orders for my blood and urine tests were sent electronically to the laboratory department, which was down the hall from my primary care doctor. My husband and I sat in the patient lobby until I was called to get my blood drawn and to give urine. When I was called to the laboratory room, I let the phlebotomist take my blood. She gave me the necessary cup for my urine. Once everything was done, my husband and I left.

It was now August and I was at my primary care office, following up on the results of my blood and urine tests. The nurse called me back to check my vitals, which included my blood pressure, temperature, pulse, and respiration. My blood pressure was elevated. I never experienced high blood pressure until now. I know it was probably high due to the severe pain I was constantly in and the worry about what was causing it. After the nurse checked and recorded my vitals, she took my husband and me to the exam room where we waited to see my doctor. Within minutes, she came in the room. After greeting us, she sat down in her chair at a small desk with a laptop sitting on it. She logged in, brought up my chart, and faced me. She gave me the blood results first. She explained to me that my inflammation levels were high, including my cholesterol.

I nodded, not surprised. "Of course my inflammation levels are elevated, because of the pain I am in. Both of my legs are inflamed. You can see how swollen they are. They also have these speckled, zigzag-looking lines on them from my thighs all the way to the tops of my knees. And they are hot when you touch them, as if they have a fever."

"Can you please roll up your pants so I can take a look?" the doctor asked.

Instead of rolling up my pants leg, I pulled them down below my knees. She looked at them and then touched them. She explained to me that both of them were inflamed.

"Can you test me for lupus?" I asked. "My half-sister and cousin both have it. They are both relatives on my dad's side."

"You would have to have symptoms in order to be tested," she replied.

"I did my research online," I persisted. "The speckled, zigzag pattern and swelling are there for a reason. On both of my cheeks, I am starting to develop a butterfly rash. And the increase in weight and the severe pain – something has to be causing all of those symptoms. I don't think it is from the sciatica. If it is lupus, I want to start the treatments ASAP. I don't want to be that one patient who wasn't tested for it because it was missed, and then receive the bad news that it is too late or it is too far gone to treat."

The doctor consulted my chart again. "Have you had an EMG on both of your legs?"

"Yes," I nodded. "I had an EMG on both of my legs years ago. It was normal."

"Alright, I am going to test you for lupus," she said. "I am also going to send orders over for an EMG and MRIs of your lower back. I want to see you back for a follow-up after I receive the results."

"Okay, I have no problem with getting an EMG and the MRIs. Is there anything else I can do for the severe pain that I am in? The medication prescribed to me by the ER doctor is not helping."

"I don't want to put you on something that might harm you," she explained. "If you could just tolerate the pain until after you do the tests and after I get the results, we can then move forward."

"Well, you are the doctor. I guess I can tolerate the pain until you get the results."

My husband and I walked out of the exam room to the nurses' station to check out. I made a follow-up appointment and was given the orders for the EMG on both of my legs and the MRIs on my lower back.

A few days later, my husband and I went to the MRI facility to do the MRIs. The radiology technician explained to me that my results would be sent to my doctor electronically. Once she was satisfied with the images, we left.

In the midst of me going back and forth to the ER and the doctor's office, I kept working. I would drive myself to and from work, 24.1 miles/45 minutes (due to rush hour traffic) every day, working from 8:30 am to 5:30 pm. I worked one-on-one with a doctor for the past 13 years.

Regardless of whether I was driving or just lying in my bed, the pain was there and it wasn't easing up. I found myself crying, day and night. I had never experienced pain like that ever in my life. Giving birth to a child was nothing compared to the pain I was having. Every day my husband would help me into a tub of hot water with alcohol and Epsom salt. I would lie in the tub until the water started getting cold. After I was done, my husband would come and help me out. Once I was dressed, I would get into our bed using a step stool because my bed was high off the floor. The pain of trying to get in our bed was two times worse than the pain I was already experiencing. My husband bought me a heating pad to use for the pain. It didn't help. He also tried an ice pack. That didn't help, either. I started using two pillows between my legs when I laid on my side and under my knees when lying on my back. For some strange reason, that eased the pain some, but not much.

Before I could do the EMG and follow-up with my primary care doctor after her requested tests, I ended up going to the ER yet again. We went back to the same one from the last time because my primary care doctor was affiliated with that ER. All of my records from her and anything I had done in her office could be uploaded on the ER doctor's systems. And, of course, it was vice versa with her. Whatever I did, it didn't decrease the pain. The pillow between my legs and under my knees stopped working. It seemed as if whenever I thought I was getting ahead of the problem, it beat me every time. It was always three steps ahead of me.

After I got checked into the ER, I was sent back to the exam room immediately to be seen by the ER doctor. It was explained to my husband and me that the reason for the prompt service was because I was recently there. It was also brought to our attention that the doctor had read my medical records from my primary care doctor and her advice to bring me back.

Once the doctor came in the room, it was the same as always: Where do you hurt? Are you doing anything different? I see you had an MRI of the lower back. The results are showing you have an L5 disc budging. It's nothing to be worried about. It doesn't require surgery.

And yet he ordered blood to be drawn and urine for testing. Once he received the results, the nurse came in and explained to my husband and me that my blood levels showed my inflammation level was extremely high and he wanted me to follow up with my primary care doctor, but wrote a prescription for more pain medications. By this time, I was pissed. Enough was enough! How can you keep giving me pain medications without knowing what the heck was wrong with me? I told my husband I was ready to go. He got up, helped me off the bed, and we left.

Chapter 5

What I couldn't understand was why in the hell these doctors couldn't figure out what was causing the excruciating pain that was interfering with my everyday life! I knew all of this wasn't in my head. I worked in the medical field. I had been working at a doctor's office for 13 years, for a neurologist and a psychiatrist. I was resuming my career to go back to college for medical school. I knew for a fact from working for these doctors that some people can become depressed and suicidal. I wasn't going to give up on what the hell was going on with me. As a young girl, I could remember all the times I got sick and missed a lot of school but I can't remember experiencing any pain like this. The pain I was experiencing wouldn't let you forget it. It was now part of my short-term and long-term memory.

After the last visit to the ER, I just lived with the pain, day by day, while not knowing what was wrong with me. Every day and night, it seemed to be getting worse. It felt as if my follow-up appointment to see my primary doctor was taking its time getting here.

On my next follow-up appointment, I saw a different doctor because my doctor was on vacation. I described to him every visit to the ER and every appointment with my regular doctor. I also explained to him that I thought I had lupus because of the symptoms I was experiencing. I told him how much everything I was going through was affecting my life. I couldn't focus on my normal daily tasks, I couldn't sleep. I told him that not knowing was the worst. How can you treat something if you don't know what you are treating? I explained to him that I wasn't going to be their guinea pig by taking different medications to treat my symptoms. That I'd never had high blood pressure until I started experiencing all of this pain. I showed him the speckled pattern on both of my legs and how inflamed they were. I told him I had a high fever and that I gained weight from the inflammation. I showed him the butterfly-looking facial rash that was on my upper cheeks and how red my face was. I took my cell phone out of my purse and showed him before and after pictures of myself so he could understand what I was telling him.

The doctor asked me, "Are you at risk of suicide or have you thought about suicide?"

"No," I told him.

"Do you think you are experiencing anxiety from everything that's being going on with you?"

"Yes," I answered, "I know I am. I am indeed human. All of this pain and not knowing what is causing it would make anyone have anxiety. Who wouldn't?"

"Looking over your blood work, I see your cholesterol is high, and of course we know why your inflammation levels are high. You tested negative for all drug levels as well as all of the STDs (sexually transmitted diseases). I am going to go look at your scans and the results from your MRI. I'll be right back." He left the room.

Minutes later, the doctor returned. He explained to me the same thing the ER doctor and my primary doctor said. He suggested for me to keep my appointments for both the EMG and the follow-up appointment that was already made prior to this appointment. He prescribed me something for my anxiety that would also help with sleep and pain. He also prescribed me something for the inflammation.

I explained to him that I didn't want to take anything that was addictive and might cause weight gain. I also told him I didn't want to be taking a lot of medications to treat my symptoms.

He put me on light duty at work until I would come back to see him after the EMG.

"Can you refer me to a rheumatologist?" I asked.

"Why do you need to see a rheumatologist?"

"I need to be further tested," I insisted. "I need to see a specialist, someone experienced with rare diseases, someone who can test me on a higher level. I know something is not right, I can feel it within my body. Something isn't right. My symptoms are beyond your expertise and I need to see someone with knowledge about everything that is going on with me since it seems as if my regular doctor and the ER doctors were guessing and playing with my health."

Before he could answer me, I explained to him how a lot of my family were misdiagnosed, which cost them their lives. He looked at me for what seemed like several minutes.

Finally, he said, "It's not going to be easy to get a referral for you to see a rheumatologist, but I will try."

I breathed a sigh of relief. "Thank you. Knowing you are going to try is better than not trying at all."

"Make sure you pick up your light duty note for work," he reminded me. "Call back in a few days to see where we stand on the referral."

"Okay, will do."

"See you at your next appointment. Have a great day."

I walked out of the exam room to the check-out desk. There, a follow-up appointment for him was made because my doctor was still going to be on vacation. My prescription was sent electronically to the pharmacy, and the nurse gave me the note to give to my boss for light duty. She explained to me that I would receive a call once they got the referral for me to see the rheumatologist.

"Okay," I said, and then left.

I waited a few days before I called to check on the referral to see the rheumatologist. The rheumatologist's office had gotten the referral but was booked solid. The next appointment for a new patient was almost two months away. The person I was talking to was a scheduler for the specialist. She told me if anyone cancelled before then, I would receive a call. I wanted to get hostile with her but didn't. I was already in pain. I didn't want to stress myself out and cause more problems.

Two weeks before my scheduled EMG, on November 24, 2013, I started experiencing a different type of pain. It felt like someone was hammering away on the bones in both of my legs. I found myself taking the pain medication two hours before my normally scheduled time. My husband was sitting in front of the computer in our room, taking an online test for his scheduled class. I quietly interrupted him and told him something wasn't right. I described the pain I was feeling and that it was causing me to become immobile. I couldn't walk. I told him to continue taking his test, and that I was going to get our youngest son to drive me to the ER.

I decided I was going to the one that was closer to the house. I didn't want to go back to the ER we had been to twice before. I was going to the one I went to when I first started experiencing this pain. At least the doctors there did more to find out what was causing the pain even though they couldn't pinpoint the exact cause. I had just gone to the other ER because my primary doctor was affiliated with that one.

At first my husband wanted to take me without finishing his online exam, but I was able to convince him to stay home and let our son take me. I explained to him that we would keep him informed about my status.

At that time, both my husband and son were taking classes towards their associate degrees. I had registered for pre-med classes and had to drop them due to the excruciating pain I was experiencing. I didn't want to start classes and then later have to drop out and throw away money because of what the outcome of my pain might be.

I went into our son's room and asked him to come take me to the ER. He changed his clothes, grabbed his wallet, and we said goodbye to my husband and left. As we got in the car, I held back the tears because I didn't want my son to see how much pain I was in. Within 30 minutes, we were pulling in to the ER parking lot.

Chapter 6

My son got out of the car and ran over to my side, opened the door, and helped me walk to the door. Once we were in, I checked in at the front with a nurse. She gave me forms to fill out, and I completed as much as I could. When I was finished, my son grabbed the forms from me and took them back to the nurse. During previous trips to the doctor or ER, my husband would help me complete the forms and I signed them.

After my son turned in the forms, I was called back immediately by the nurse. She took my vitals, and as always, everything was elevated.

"Your blood pressure, temperature, pulse and respiration are high," the nurse commented. "Are you on any medications for the high blood pressure? Have you taken anything for this fever?"

"Yes, I am on medication for the high blood pressure," I told her. "As for the fever, I didn't know it was high."

The nurse jotted something down on my chart. "I am going to ask the doctor if I can give you something for the fever. I see here that you came in with severe pain in both legs and lower back."

"Yes, I was also here in 2005 for the same thing I am experiencing now. I have seen my primary care doctor and been twice to the ER that she is affiliated with in regards to this matter, but I am not getting any better. They seem as if they don't know what they're doing."

"I will be right back after I talk to the doctor about something for this high temperature."

The nurse left the room. I sat there patiently, but in pain, waiting for her to return. My son was texting his dad and brother with an update.

The nurse came back into the room. "I have two Tylenols and a small cup of water to give you for the fever."

"Thank you," I said.

I took the Tylenols and drank the water. Then the nurse asked us to follow her. We didn't go back to the patient waiting area, but rather into an exam room. The nurse asked me to have a seat on the bed or to lie down, if I preferred. She told me the doctor would be in shortly. I thanked her as she was leaving the room.

My son texted my husband and my oldest son again, informing them that we were now in an exam room, waiting to see the doctor. Shortly after, the ER doctor walked in.

"Good evening," she said. "I have read your chart and was able to pull up your records from 2005. Thank you for letting us know you were here back then with the same problem."

"No problem. I know from experience, it's always best to compare previous medical records. Especially, if it's similar to the problem before. And it is."

"Can you describe to me the pain you are in and show me where you are hurting?"

"I am hurting in my lower back," I told her. "The pain is moving from my lower back around to the front of my inner thighs, down to my knees. But the pain in both of my legs doesn't hurt at the same time. Instead, it hurts in one of my upper legs towards my inner thigh and travels down to the top of my knee. The pain never goes below my knees. Then the pain would stop hurting in that leg and move to the other leg, hurting the exact same way."

"Not including 2005, when did this new pain reoccur? Did it hurt every day until today?"

"After I was discharged from here in 2005, I had an EMG by one of the neurologists I worked for. The test came back normal. After the days, weeks, months and years went by, I didn't have the pain again until July 4, 2013. I've tried every home remedy. I have gone back and forth to my primary care doctor as well as the hospital she is affiliated with. Because of this excruciating pain, I now have hypertension and anxiety. I am losing sleep every night and I am on light duty at work. The doctors I've seen can't make a diagnosis. So, they wanted to give me medications for every symptom I am having, but I told all of them. I wasn't a guinea pig. Both of my legs are inflamed. It feels as if they have a fever. I have speckled-looking patterns on both of my legs. In the past few weeks, I gained weight and I am sure it's the inflammation in my legs."

"Let me take a look at your legs," the doctor said. "Before I do so, why don't you change into a gown? What is your son's name? Can you please step out so your mother can change and I can examine her? You don't have to go far, just wait outside the curtain. I'll let you know when you can return. Thank you."

"Sure, no problem," my son said. "Mom, I'll be right outside. Love you."

"Love you, too," I responded.

The doctor smiled with approval. "He is such a great son to be here at the hospital with you."

"Yes, he is," I answered in response to the doctor's comment. "Both of my sons are. My husband is, too. I asked him to stay home because he was taking his midterms online. He's been going back and forth to the ER and appointments with me. He really wanted to come but I assured him I would be okay. Plus, my son is very responsible and he has been texting his dad and his brother with updates on my status."

After my son left the room, the doctor closed the curtain on my side of the area and handed me two gowns, one to put on that tied in the back, and one to put on over it that opened in the front.

After I got dressed, the doctor helped me back on the bed. She asked me to lie on my back while she examined me. She looked into my ears, nose and mouth. Next, she checked my neck with her fingers. Then she asked me to cough while she listened to my throat with the stethoscope. She grabbed me by the hand and forearm and helped me sit up. She lifted my gowns, placed the stethoscope on my back and asked me to cough again. She pulled my gowns back down and lifted them in the front to look at my legs. She looked at me with a puzzled expression on her face. She touched both of my legs and looked at me again.

"Can you feel my hands?" she asked.

"Yes," I said.

The doctor moved her hands. "Which leg or legs am I touching?"

"Both," I answered.

"They are indeed swollen with quite a bit of inflammation, and they are hot to the touch. Did you fall or were you involved in an accident?"

I shook my head. "No, I haven't fallen nor been involved in an accident."

"Point and show me where you hurt," the doctor instructed.

I pointed to the area of my lower back, all around to my inner thighs, and down to the tops of my knees.

The doctor consulted my chart again. "I see here on your forms that there's a history of lupus on your father's side," she said. "Have you been tested for lupus?"

"Yes, after I asked and convinced my primary care doctor, she finally checked some levels for me."

"What were the results?" she asked.

"It showed positive, speckled and 80."

"I see the name of the ER and the names of the doctors you have seen in the previous months. I am going to start by ordering some tests. This is my first time seeing you and just by looking at you, I know you are in severe pain, and looking at your body, it's obvious something is wrong."

"Okay, and thank you," I said.

"I am going to give you something for the pain, order some blood, and get a couple of scans."

"Okay."

"I am looking at a list of medications you wrote down," she added. "Are these your current medications you are taking? Has any of it helped at all?"

"Yes, I have included current medications I am taking, both prescribed and over-the-counter. And no, they are not helping."

The doctor smiled apologetically. "I am sorry, because if they were, you wouldn't be here. I see you are allergic to doxycycline. What was the reaction?"

"It causes nausea and dizziness. I get so sick to the stomach that I throw up."

"I am going to have the nurse bring you something for the pain and get some blood. I am going to call the radiology department to see if they could come get you right away as well. You marked off that you are not pregnant?"

"Yes," I nodded in the direction where my son went, "he's my youngest son and he's in college. No more children for me."

"I am going to let them know that you are a high risk for falling. You need to be in a wheelchair and need supervision when you are mobile. I am going to tell your son he can come back in with you."

"Thank you," I said as she left the room.

Within minutes, my son returned to the closed area where I was lying down. Not long after that, the nurse came in with pain medication and a small cup of water. After I took the medication, she drew my blood, made sure I was comfortable, and left.

"Mom, what did the doctor say?" my son asked.

"She is ordering different blood tests and getting some scans of my back. She is trying to make a diagnosis."

"I am going to text dad and my brother to let them know what is going on now. They texted me while the doctor was in examining you."

I lay there, hoping and praying that this doctor could find out what was causing this excruciating pain, because at this point, I was sick and tired of being sick and tired.

Chapter 7

My prayers were interrupted by a male radiology technician. He came in with a wheelchair to take me to the radiology room.

"Hello," he said. "Can I see your wrist bands to make sure I am getting the right patient?"

I raised my hand towards him so he could take a look at my identification bands.

"Okay, I have the right patient," he said with a friendly smile. "I am going to help you sit up and then help you get in the wheelchair. But first, let me lock the wheels so the chair won't move."

He helped me out of the bed onto my two feet, and then into the wheelchair. He unlocked the wheelchair and rolled me out, telling my son to follow. Once we got to the radiology room, the technician locked the wheelchair, helped me onto the extremely cold table, and began the scans. Just lying there on my back seemed to take forever. I wanted him to be finished, like now. Finally, he was done. He helped me back into the wheelchair, then told me he needed to look at the films to make sure they were okay. The scans were to his satisfaction. He unlocked the wheelchair and wheeled me back to the area I was in, my son following. The technician locked the wheelchair and helped me back into the bed.

"I hope you start feeling better," he said. "The doctor will be receiving the results of the scans shortly. Have a nice night."

"Thank you."

Shortly after the radiology technician left, the doctor came back in.

"How are you feeling now after taking the pain medications?" she enquired.

I shook my head. "There is no change! I feel the same."

"Really?" She sounded surprised. "That should have helped with the pain."

"No, it did not. I feel as if I still have a fever as well."

"Let me check your temperature." After taking my temperature and reading the measurement, the doctor exclaimed, "It is still high! It is higher than when you first came in. It is 102.9. I am going to call the head ER doctor and get some advice. I may have to admit you. Will that be alright with you?"

I nodded wearily. "I just want the pain to go away. I am tired of hurting. I don't care if you admit me! Just make the pain go away." By that time, the tears were running down my face at full force. I looked over at my son, who had his hand over his mouth. I could tell he was hurting inside for me and for what I'd been going through.

"Please give me a second," the doctor said, and left the room.

I lay there, trying to stop my tears, but they were coming down, out of my control. I looked over at my son, and saw his fingers moving over his phone at a rapid rate. I was sure he was texting his dad and brother. I asked him to get me my phone from out of my purse. I pushed the button to turn it on to try and call my husband, but the phone turned off. I tried again to turn it on, but it turned off again. I gave my phone to my son and explained to him what was going on with it. He did several things to it, then told me he thought it had a virus because it wouldn't stay on and it was at full charge. I shook my head and closed my eyes. I prayed, asking to please stop the pain for my birthday. I didn't want anything else. All I wanted was the pain to stop, to go away. I wiped my face and opened my eyes because I heard voices as they got closer to me. It was the doctor and the nurse.

The doctor told us, "I have talked to the head ER doctor. Your scans only show the bulging disc. It is the same from 2005. We know that is not the reason you are in so much pain. We do not want to release you until we find the cause. It is our job as doctors to make sure our patients are taken care of when they come to the ER. My shift is coming to an end, so he has suggested we start an IV and give you morphine through the IV for pain. He has also advised me to admit you to see if we can get to the bottom of this. I have called the Admissions department to get you a room ready so we can transport you."

"Okay," I said wearily, "if that's what it takes to get to the bottom of this and stop this pain."

"Mom," my son said, looking up from his phone, "Dad and my brother are on their way up here. My brother just texted me. They are pulling into the parking lot. I am going to go meet them at the door so I can show them where you are."

"Okay," I told him, and he left the room.

The doctor smiled. "Where can I get a son like yours? He is just a sweetheart!"

"Thank you. He gets it from both his mother and father. His brother is also like him."

"Well you and your husband have raised great sons."

I smiled proudly.

"The nurse is getting ready to hook you up to the IV and give you the first dosage of the morphine. We will be administering the morphine every four hours for pain. I am going to wait until you have been transported to your new room and are settled before I end my shift."

The nurse finished inserting the needle for my IV and pushed the first dosage of the morphine through. I immediately felt some relief from the excruciating pain. I looked over at the clock. It was 12:00 am on November 25, 2013. It was my birthday. I turned thirty-nine and got my wish for my birthday. Tears ran down my face fast. But this time, they weren't tears of pain, they were tears of joy! Tears of relief! After four months, I finally had some relief. As I was wiping my face, my husband

35

and both of our sons walked in. My husband kissed me and wished me a happy birthday. The doctor and nurse looked at me with big smiles on their faces. They knew then my tears were of joy. My sons kissed me on my cheek and told me happy birthday.

"You are in the hospital for your birthday," the doctor commented. "That's not right."

I waved my hand dismissively. "No, it is alright. I got my wish."

"Not in all of that pain, huh?" my husband said.

"Nope, some but not like before."

My oldest son grinned at me. "That's good to hear, Mom."

"Yes, it is."

"You are admitting her. What is the next step for her?" my husband asked.

"We are trying to find out the cause of the pain," the doctor explained. "I was advised by the head ER doctor to not release her until we found out."

My husband nodded. "That's good to hear. She has been through so much. I have never seen her like this. She has gone from an energetic person who always kept a smile on her face, to this."

"That's another reason why we don't want to discharge her: because she is in a lot of pain. Any person, including me, could see she is in a lot of pain. Her entire face is red. She is running a 102.9 temperature, and both of her legs are inflamed and hot to the touch. She has a history of whatever is going on."

"Yes, I know," said my husband. "She was admitted here back in 2005. The doctors back then ran a lot of tests on her but still couldn't make a diagnosis. What I can't understand is, why this year? Why skip years? It went from 2005 to now 2013. That's eight years later."

The doctor shook her head. "I don't know. If it was me treating her, I would have kept her until I found out the cause. It is something causing her to be in all of this pain and causing her to have such a high temperature. Her body is trying to fight something, but what, I have no clue."

"Thank you for trying to help her. For once in several months she is not suffering with a lot of pain."

"Doctor, her room is ready," said the nurse. "They are on the way to transport her."

"Thank you," the doctor answered. "I will be writing up her orders in her chart. That way, the covering doctor will know what to expect. It was nice talking to you and treating your wife. I can say, I have never seen a case like hers. I wish I could stay and treat her until I find out the cause, but I can't; it's out of my control now."

"I am still thankful for your efforts and for giving her some relief."

"They are here to transport her. I wish you all well. Please continue to lead your sons in the right direction."

"Thank you so much for everything you have done for me," I told the doctor. "I also wish you well. Don't ever stop being you. You are that one doctor who puts herself in others' shoes and has a caring heart. I know you are not in your profession for the money, and I admire you for that."

"Thank you. I hope you have a wonderful birthday despite being in the hospital."

And she was gone.

Chapter 8

"Boys, it's late, you can go ahead and go home," I told my sons. "Call your dad when you get home so we know you two are home and safe."

They both kissed me on the cheek, told me happy birthday again, told me they loved me. I could see in our sons' eyes they were worried and concerned about me. I reassured them I wasn't going to give up, I wasn't going to let whatever this was get the very best of me and I was going to fight with everything within me. They both told me they loved me again and left.

The porters helped me into the wheelchair, transported me to my new room, and carefully helped me on the bed. They arranged my IV so I wouldn't accidently pull it out, made sure I was comfortable, and left.

I gave my husband my cell phone and told him it was dead.

"Everyone is texting me, checking on you," my husband told me. "I told them you have been admitted into the hospital."

"Alright. Can I see your phone?"

"You should go on Facebook and let them know your status," he suggested.

"Okay, I will do it now."

Using my husband's phone, I logged in to Facebook and updated my status. I gave a brief summary of what was going on with me for the past 72 hours and logged out. As I was returning my husband's cell phone back to him, the doctor walked in.

"Good early morning!" he said. "Can you please explain to me why you are here? I've read your chart but I want to hear it from you."

I proceeded to explain. "I have been experiencing excruciating pain in both of my legs from my lower back around to the front of my right inner thigh, down to the tops of my knees. It doesn't hurt in both of my legs at the same time. It's at different times. The pain feels like someone is drilling into my lower back and leg. At the moment it's hurting in my right leg. When my left leg begins to hurt, my right leg will stop hurting."

"When did all this start?" asked the doctor.

"In 2005, I was admitted in this hospital with the same symptoms. The doctors ordered numerous diagnostic tests on me. They took a tremendous amount of blood, and ordered many scans of my lower back, legs and knees. They also did several Dopplers as well. I was in the hospital for a week. I was discharged without being diagnosed."

"Were you involved in an accident or did you fall?"

"No," I answered.

"I read in your chart you have been following up with your primary care physician and one of her colleagues, and have been to the ER twice. Can you explain to me what your primary care physician and the emergency room physicians did?"

"They also took a lot of blood from me and took scans of my lower back," I said. "They only came up with a sciatica nerve and bulging discs. I had to convince my primary doctor to test me for lupus."

"Why do you think it is lupus?"

"I think it's a possibility it could be lupus, because both my sister and my cousin have lupus. I did some research myself on the signs and symptoms of lupus. I have swelling in both of my upper legs all the way down to the ends of my knees. I also have swelling in my inner thighs that is constantly hot as if they have a fever. I have speckled patterns on both of my legs that can come from inflammation. I researched the pattern and it is very similar to livedo reticularis (which can be due to spasms of the blood vessels, a serious underlying condition, such as vascular disease, endocrine disorder, or a rheumatologic disease such as lupus). I started noticing a butterfly rash forming on my cheeks to the center of my nose. I have also picked up weight with all of this inflammation. I keep a high temperature. I am not sure if it is from the pain. I do know inflammation causes pain and fluid, which causes weight gain."

"Yes, inflammation does cause weight gain due to the water," said the doctor. "Can I please take a look at the speckled pattern on your legs and the rash on your face?"

I pulled the bed spread and sheets off my legs. Next, I pulled up the hospital gown so he could take a look. He noticed the purple speckled patterns on both of my inflamed legs. He grabbed two medical gloves out of the box and put them on. He touched both of my legs. He looked at me with a confused, puzzled expression on his face.

"How long did you say you had this on both of your legs?"

"Since July when all of the pain came back."

"Four months?" he asked.

"Yes."

The doctor began looking at the butterfly rash on my face. "When did this start appearing on your face? I can definitely see what you are talking about."

"I started noticing it right after the pain, after my legs became inflamed," I told him.

My husband spoke up. "I am tired of seeing my wife in all of this pain. She has been through so much. She is losing sleep. She has seen doctor after doctor and had test after test. Something has to give. Someone needs to tell us why she is constantly in so much pain."

"I am going to do everything I can to find out her primary diagnosis," answered the doctor. "She has given me enough to go by. I am going to test her for lupus and anything else that may be the cause of all of her symptoms. I am also going to get an MRI."

"She is claustrophobic," my husband said. "She will need something to sedate her."

"No problem. Now, from one to ten, what is your pain level?"

"I'd rather go through natural child birth without pain medication instead of having this pain!" I exclaimed.

The doctor nodded. "That is some pain. I see they have been giving you morphine in your IV every four hours for the pain. I am going to start you on Solu-Medrol."

"That is a steroid," I said. "It is given to patients with a diagnosis of multiple sclerosis."

"Yes it is!" The doctor looked impressed. "Oh, that's right. You work for a neurologist."

"Yes!" I answered.

"It will be administered into your IV several times with different dosages. It will be given to you to treat the pain. Your pain level will drop tremendously. Do you have any questions?"

"I am sensitive to medications," I informed him, "so hopefully the Solu-Medrol won't make me sick."

"If so, ring for the nurse and let them know. I am going to flag your chart just in case."

"Thank you."

"Thanks for your help," my husband added.

"How long do you think I will be here?" I asked the doctor.

"Hopefully three days max. Now, I am going to go and get the medication. I will be right back with one of the nurses."

The doctor left the room. My husband's cell phone started ringing. He looked at his phone before answering it. It was my mother calling to check on me. My husband answered the call and began explaining to her what the doctor was going to do."

I lay in the bed, staring at the television. I had no idea what was on. I needed to go to the bathroom but was afraid to move. My husband was still on his phone talking to my mother. All of a sudden there was a knock at the door, and then it opened. It was a radiology technician coming to get me for my scans.

"Hello, can I check your wrist band to make sure I have the right patient?"

My husband had finished talking to my mother and now addressed the technician. "Did you bring something for her to take before the MRI? She is claustrophobic!"

"No, I don't administer medications," the technician said. "The doctor or nurse is supposed to give the patient the medication at least 30 minutes before the scan."

"The doctor just left," responded my husband. "He hasn't been back. You will need to come back after she takes the medication."

"I have orders to take her now."

"I should be okay," I said. "I will just not think about being in that big, closed tube."

My husband was insistent. "No, he just needs to come back later."

I sighed. "I am going to go ahead and get it over with. How many scans is it?"

"It's just one scan."

I eased out of the bed and onto the floor. I slowly walked over and sat down in the wheelchair. The radiology technician unlocked the wheelchair and pushed me out of the room, down the hallway to the radiology room. Once we were in the room, the technician locked the wheelchair, helped me out of it, and held my arm until I got onto the cold, flat, iron table. I knew for sure that thing was freezing. (It is always cold in the radiology rooms. I am assuming it is because of the film they use for the images.) The radiology technician helped me onto the freezing metal table, then went into the control room. He was giving me instructions when he was interrupted by a call. By the sound of his voice and the look on his face, he was scared. He walked back over to me.

"We are not going to do the scan," he told me. "The doctor asked me to bring you back to the room."

"I wonder why? That's never happened to me. I wonder what that is about."

"I have no idea," the technician answered.

The radiology technician helped me off the freezing cold table and back into the wheelchair. He unlocked the wheels and pushed me out of the radiology room up the hall and back into my room.

Chapter 9

The radiology technician opened the door and wheeled me towards the bed. He locked the wheelchair and helped me out, but I stopped him in his tracks. I still had to go to the bathroom. After all of this time, I hadn't had a chance to go. I slowly walked to the bathroom door, opened it and went in. Once I was finished, I washed my hands and slowly walked out and closed the door. The head of the bed wasn't far from the bathroom door. When I got to the bed, my husband helped me onto the bed and made sure I was comfortable before he sat back down. Not too long after that, there was a knock on the door and then it opened. The doctor entered with a nurse behind him.

"I canceled your MRI," the doctor explained. "If it showed normal, I would have to release you. I am going to wait for the results to come back on your blood and go from there. But in the meantime, I am going to go ahead and start your first dose of your Solu-Medrol. It's going to start working within minutes. It should decrease your pain and help you get some sleep."

"I am glad you cancelled her MRI," said my husband. "When the guy came in to get her for the test, I explained to him that she is claustrophobic and will need something to help sedate her. He did not pay me any attention. He said he was doing what was requested."

The doctor shook his head. "It was on the top of her chart in big red letters that she is claustrophobic. He knew better not to get her until she was sedated."

"I thought so. I didn't say anything else because my wife said it was okay and she wanted it to be over with."

"I will be calling the radiology department after I finish with your first dosage of the Solu-Medrol," the doctor assured us.

The nurse and the doctor put on gloves, then she handed him the alcohol swab and the medication vial. He disinfected the top of the medication vial, inserted the needle, and pulled on the needle handle until all of the medication was in the syringe. He then inserted the needle into the IV tube and slowly pushed the medication into my IV.

"You are going to feel the medication as it enters your vein," advised the doctor. "Let me know what you are feeling."

"I can feel a warm sensation. It is making me feel as if I am in a trance, more like a daze. I feel light."

"Okay, that is normal. I am almost done."

Suddenly I realized something. "I don't feel any pain! It's gone!"

"Really?" My husband was astonished. "You are not hurting?"

"Nope, I feel nothing."

"I am all done. Please keep an eye on her," the doctor told my husband. "Call the nurses' station if you need to."

"Will do, thank you."

I looked up at the doctor. "Thank you doctor! After over four months, I am pain-free."

"That's what I needed to hear," he smiled. "The nurse is going to go ahead and get some blood from you so I can see if there are any abnormalities."

"Okay, thanks again!" I called, as he turned to leave.

The nurse approached the side of my bed. "I have everything prepared so we can get this over with. But before I do, are you feeling alright?"

"Yes, you can go ahead and draw the blood."

The nurse used several tubes with different colored tops that varied in size. She filled each tube up with my blood. I thought she wasn't going to ever finish. She filled at least twelve tubes. Once the nurse was done, she cleaned up her mess by putting everything in the proper containers. She asked us to buzz the nurses' station if we needed anything.

"How are you feeling?" my husband asked.

"I am not in pain. Just feeling light."

He smiled at me. "I am assuming that's a good thing."

"Yes!"

"That's good to know."

I paused for a moment, then clapped my hand over my mouth. "I am starting to feel sick!"

"The button for the nurse is right next to you. Go ahead and push it!"

"I can't hold it! I need to go to the bathroom!"

My husband jumped up. "Let me help you!"

Before my husband came to the side of the bed that was the closest to the bathroom door, I jumped out of the bed, ran to the bathroom, kneeled down in front of the toilet and it was all over. I threw up so much my head and stomach started hurting. My husband stood by the bathroom door to make sure I was alright. Once I was done, I went over to the sink, brushed my teeth using a new, unopened toothbrush and travel-sized toothpaste, and washed my face. When I was done, I walked out of the bathroom and got back in the bed. My husband looked at me and I looked at him.

"Do you realize you jumped out of the bed and literally ran to the bathroom?" he asked.

I grimaced. "I was feeling really nauseous and couldn't keep it down. I had to go. If not, it would have gotten very messy in here."

"The medicine really works. Are you still feeling sick?"

"Yes, I am going to push the button for the nurses' station. I need something to settle my stomach."

I pushed the button and someone else answered. It wasn't the nurse that came in with the doctor.

"Hello!" the nurse's voice called out. "How may I help you?"

"I am feeling sick from the Solu-Medrol," I answered. "I've already thrown up. Can I please have something for this nausea?"

"Yes, I'll be right there."

"Thank you."

I lay there in that bed with the sheet over my head, trying to shake the sick feeling. I was thankful to not be in pain but now I felt sick to my stomach. The feeling was like being on a roller coaster going straight down at a rapid speed.

My husband stood up from the recliner he was sitting in, got a small towel out the bathroom, and wet it with cold water. He pulled the sheet slightly off my face and placed the towel on my forehead.

There was a knock at the door. It opened and the nurse came in with a pre-filled syringe.

"Hello," she said. "I will be taking care of you for the next twelve hours. I have brought something to stop the nausea."

The nurse took a look at my hospital wrist bands to make sure I was the right patient. She put on a pair of gloves, wiped the tube on my IV with an alcohol swab, stuck a needle into the tube, and slightly pushed the medication in until the syringe was empty. She threw the syringe and the alcohol swab in their respective biohazard containers.

"The medicine should kick in within ten minutes," the nurse said. "How are you feeling right now?"

"I feel light-headed," I answered.

"That is one of the side effects of the nausea medication. It will most likely put you to sleep."

"That's a good thing," said my husband. "She hasn't had a good night's sleep for months. Well, me and her both. When she's hurting and can't sleep, I can't sleep."

"How long have you been hurting?" the nurse asked me.

"Four months."

She looked surprised. "They haven't found out what is causing the pain?"

"No!" exclaimed my husband. "It's been a long road for her. Hopefully, the doctor here will be able to tell us something."

The nurse consulted my chart. "I see he's ordered a lot of blood tests. Hopefully, the doctor will have an answer to the problem. I am going to be close by so if you need anything, please buzz the nurses' station. They should be bringing breakfast in. Try to eat a little."

"I will try, and thank you." I said to her.

Before I knew it, I was asleep.

It seemed as if I was asleep for days; I almost forgot what it felt like to sleep. It had been four months since I had a good night's sleep. The pain was so bad I couldn't take a nap even if I wanted to. It didn't matter if I slept on my back, my side, on the couch, in a chair, or in my bed, that pain didn't let me sleep.

I woke up to someone touching me. It was the doctor.

"Hello," he said, "I didn't mean to wake you and disturb your sleep. I have to give you the second dose of the Solu-Medrol. We have to be persistent. How are you feeling?"

"I am not in all of that pain like I was before," I commented. "I am feeling more numb than anything. I am feeling somewhat different now after you injected the medication."

"Is that a bad thing or a good thing?"

"It's a good thing but I am starting to feel a little queasy."

"I am going to have the nurse bring the nausea medication and have her administer it before you start feeling worse," said the doctor. "In the meantime, try to get some more rest before your next scheduled dose."

"Thank you," I said.

"Besides feeling nauseous from the first dose of the Solu-Medrol, how did you feel?"

"She ran to the bathroom," my husband answered for me.

"What do you mean by ran?"

"She couldn't hold the nausea any longer. She had to go throw up. She couldn't wait for me to help her out of the bed and to the bathroom so she jumped out of the bed and ran into the bathroom."

The doctor's eyebrows raised. "That's something."

"I thought the same thing," said my husband.

"We're making progress," the doctor assured us. "Now the question is, what's causing all of the pain, inflammation, and high temperature? Hopefully, I will have answers by tomorrow morning. By the way, I saw the people from the cafeteria. They should be bringing your breakfast. Make sure you try and eat something."

"I will," I said.

As the doctor was leaving the room, a young girl spoke to him as she was entering. She was from the hospital cafeteria and she carried a tray with food, milk, orange juice, and silverware. She pulled the bedside tray to me and placed the food tray on it. My husband pushed the button on the bed to raise my head up. I sat up in the bed as if I was going to eat the food, but the way I was feeling, I just knew that wasn't going to happen. The feeling of nausea isn't pleasant. Just smelling the food on the tray made me sick to the stomach. As the young girl was leaving the room, she told us to push the tray out of the way when we were done, and someone would be in later to get it.

"Will do," my husband called after her.

I looked at the tray of food with a grimace. "I don't want to eat. I am feeling very nauseous with the food in front of me. Can you please move it out of the way?"

"The doctor wants you to eat something," my husband protested.

"I will try after the nurse gives me something for the nausea. I wish she would come already! I am getting that feeling again as if I have to throw up."

After I said that, the nurse entered the room with the prefilled syringe.

"I am sorry it took me so long," she apologized. "I had to tend to a patient a few doors down from you and I had to set up the patient in the room next to you. Please make sure you lock the door that accesses the bathroom and please use caution. If that door is not locked, anyone from the other room can walk into your room."

"Thank you for letting us know," said my husband. "I will make sure we keep that door locked."

"I am going to administer the nausea medication." The nurse slowly pushed the medication into my IV. Once she was finished, she disposed of the syringe and alcohol pad. She checked my blood pressure, temperature, pulse, and respiration. She noticed I had an elevated temperature. "Your temperature is high. I am going to go and get you something to bring it down. I see they brought your breakfast in to you. Have you tried eating any of it?"

"No, I started feeling really sick from the smell of the food. I asked my husband to put it to the side for now. Once the nausea medication kicks in, I'll try to eat some. But right now, I am feeling sick to my stomach."

"Okay, the medication should start working within minutes," the nurse said. "I am going to go and get you something for this elevated temperature. I will be right back."

The nurse left the room to go and get me something for the high fever. It just seemed so unreal with everything going on with me. I lay in the bed, rocking back and forth, trying to keep myself from feeling sick and throwing up. My husband offered me water, a cold towel, soda, and crackers to settle my stomach. Just hearing him saying those things was making it worse.

Finally, the nurse came in with two Motrins for the fever. She opened up the package and gave the tablets to me with a small cup of water. "There you go. The medication should start working within minutes. Have you tried to eat anything since I left?"

"No, just smelling the food is making me sick."

"I understand. Try to eat a little, even if it's just a couple of spoonfuls. You don't have to eat it all."

I looked at the food tray. "I will try, but I am not going to make you any promises."

"I will make sure she tries to eat something," added my husband. "She just may go to sleep because after her first dose of the nausea medication, within minutes, she was asleep."

"Okay, no problem," the nurse said. "Has she tried drinking water or a

Sprite?"

"I offered a cold towel, water, soda, and crackers, but she didn't want it."

"Okay, I will be back in here in an hour to check her vitals. If she needs anything, please call the nurses' station." The nurse walked towards the door and exited the room.

My husband stood up. "I am going to go see if I can find some place to buy a Sprite. You need to drink something besides that IV with those fluids going into your veins. If you are asleep when I return, I will just wait until you wake up to give it to you. You have been missing out on so much sleep, I refuse to wake you. I will be right back."

He kissed me on my forehead and walked out of the room. Within minutes, I felt sleep coming on. Next thing I knew, I was asleep.

Chapter 10

I woke up to the door closing behind me. I looked over to my right; my husband was asleep on the pull-out couch that was next to me. It wasn't him in the bathroom, so I assumed it was the patient that was in the room next to me.

My husband looked so peaceful sleeping, I refused to wake him. He had been losing sleep, too. Even when I dosed off, he didn't sleep. Most of the time I would catch him nodding off but not for long.

I couldn't tell if it was still day or night because the room didn't have a window. I looked up at the television; an episode of Sanford and Son was on. So I knew then it was dark outside, nighttime. I had slept the entire day away. I looked over to the left of me and there was a tray of food and beverages on it. It was something different from earlier. This morning when the girl brought the breakfast food, it included milk and juice. There was no milk carton nor juice carton on it. It looked like a cup of tea. My stomach started growling. I looked over at my husband, but he was still asleep. I had to go to the bathroom. I thought to myself, should I wake him or try to go on my own? I no longer felt pain nor nausea. So I tried easing out of the bed to go to the bathroom, which was right behind me.

My husband stirred. "Baby, do you need to go to the bathroom?"

"Yes, I was going to go by myself," I said.

"No," he protested. "I am going to help you. I don't want you to fall."

"I think I will be alright!"

"No, I am helping you," insisted my husband, standing up. "How are you feeling? How long have you been up?"

I gave in. "Alright, if you insist on helping me. I am feeling alright. I am not in any pain and I've been awake about five minutes. I heard the door close in the bathroom, that's why I am awake."

"That's right, the nurse did say earlier that someone was in the room next to us and to keep the door locked because we share the same bathroom."

My husband came around to the side of the bed where my IV was and helped me out of the bed. He slowly walked me into the bathroom, covered the toilet seat with a protective seat cover, and walked back into the hospital room, standing there until I was finished. After I washed my hands, he escorted me back to bed, making sure I was propped up comfortably. After locking the door that accessed the bathroom, he brought me the cart with the tray of food and prepared some tea, then asked me to eat.

"What are you going to eat?" I asked my husband.

"I am going to leave once you are comfortable. I am going to go to the house and get us a few things for a couple of nights. I will then stop and get myself something to eat."

"If you want to, you can go ahead and leave now," I told him. "Just make sure the remote to the television and the call button is near me just in case I need assistance."

"Do you want to drink the soda I got you earlier?" he asked. "I can go to the nurses' station and get you a cup of ice."

"Yes, please."

My husband left the room to get me a cup of ice for my soda. I started eating some of the green beans that were on the plate. I immediately started feeling sick to my stomach. I pushed the cart that had the plate on it away from me. My husband walked back in the room with a cup full of ice. He poured some of the soda in the cup and handed it to me. He noticed the cart was moved.

"What, you still can't eat?"

"No," I muttered. "I tried eating some of the green beans and I immediately started feeling sick to my stomach."

"I shouldn't leave you alone. I'll wait until tomorrow and go then."

"No, I will be alright," I told him. "I will just sip on this Sprite since it's not making me sick. Go ahead and leave. I need to change."

"I should call the boys and ask them to bring some stuff."

"No, go ahead and go. I will be alright."

I finally convinced him to leave and go to the house. Our house wasn't far from the hospital. He needed to leave anyway because he needed to get him something to eat.

After he left, I kept sipping on the cold Sprite. It went straight down because I hadn't eaten anything and it was already nighttime. It really helped calm my stomach. The door opened and the nurse came in.

"Well, good evening!" she greeted me. "How are you feeling?"

"Hello, I am doing fine."

"I see you are drinking something. That's wonderful!" she said encouragingly.

"Yes, my husband got me a Sprite. I was asleep when he came back so he went and got a cup of ice so I could drink it."

"You have a wonderful husband," commented the nurse.

I smiled. "Thank you and yes, he is the best."

"I am going to check your vitals now."

The nurse checked my blood pressure. It was okay. She then checked my pulse, respiration, and temperature. Everything was okay. She looked at my IV bags and they were half full. "Were you able to eat anything?"

"No, I tried eating some green beans and it immediately started making me sick. That's when my husband went and got some ice for the Sprite. It calmed my stomach. I am no longer feeling sick."

The nurse nodded. "Okay, at least you tried. Are you finished with the tray?"

"Yes, I am."

"I will take it out with me when I leave. Your vitals are fine. Is there anything you need before I go?"

"No, I am okay," I answered. "I am just going to sip on this soda."

"Okay, I will be back in an hour to give you your next dose of the Solu-Medrol."

The nurse left the room. I just stayed sitting up in the bed, sipping on my soda. It seemed like the best soda I had ever tasted. I couldn't help but to think to myself, what a birthday gift. I asked to be pain-free for my birthday, and here it was, November 25, 2013, my birthday. Well, birthday night, since this day was almost over. I started changing the channels on the television because I was trying to ignore my inner thoughts. Just to be lying here, thinking about how long I had been in pain. The thought of me being diagnosed with cancer, lupus, or any other type of long-term, fatal illness had my mind all over the place.

My thoughts were interrupted by my urge to go to the bathroom. I thought to myself, should I get up and take a chance and go to the bathroom by myself, or should I call the nurses' station to inform them I needed to go? The urge to go to the bathroom became more intense. Right before I got ready to push the button for the nurses' station, the door of the room slowly opened. It was my husband coming in. He was carrying a duffle bag, including several shopping bags and food. The smell of the food made my stomach growl and my mouth water.

"How are you feeling?" he enquired.

"I need to go to the bathroom. I was about to call the nurses' station when you came in."

"Okay, let me help you. Did anyone come in to check on you while I was gone?"

I nodded. "Yes, the nurse came in and checked my vitals. Everything was normal."

"That's good to know. Hopefully, they can tell us tomorrow the primary diagnosis that has been causing you to be in so much pain."

"Yes, I am hoping so."

My husband helped me to the bathroom, then escorted me back to the bed when I was done. He made sure I was cozy and comfortable in the bed. "I was going to get Chinese food but they were already closed. So, McDonald's it is."

"I didn't realize it was that late," I said.

"Yes, it's going on 11:00pm."

My husband pulled the cart over to me, grabbed the McDonald's bag, and placed a fish sandwich on it, including a medium fries. He grabbed the cup I was drinking out of and threw it in the trash, then left the room. I grabbed the fish sandwich, opened it, and took a bite. It was so good, or I was just so hungry because I hadn't eaten in almost 24 hours. I then took a fry and stuffed it into my mouth. The door opened and my husband came in with a cup filled with ice.

"I see you are eating," he said, beaming at me. "I figured you would be hungry when I got back and that's why I got you something."

"Yes, I am. I didn't eat any of the food they brought in. I couldn't. The nausea wouldn't let me."

"Did you drink all of the Sprite I bought you earlier?"

"Yes," I nodded. "The nurse threw the bottle out when she took the tray away."

"That's good to know."

He sat down on the chair, got his food, and started eating. I gave him the remote to the television. Next thing we knew, someone knocked on the door and came in. It was our friends and their two children. They stopped by to bring me my birthday gift and some balloons. They couldn't believe I was in the hospital. They were on their way to our house when she noticed my son's status on Facebook, stating I was in the hospital. She immediately texted him and caught up on what was going on. She got the name of the hospital and now here they were. She explained to us that the nurse at the front let them come to my room after visiting hours since it was my birthday. She explained to me how the nurse didn't know it was my birthday and let them go back. They stayed for a while and then left.

After our friends left my room, I started feeling sleepy. I got comfortable in the bed and started dozing off when the door opened. It was my doctor and of course I knew what time it was.

"I am going to give you the next dose of the Solu-Medrol. But before I do, I am going to give you a dose of the nausea medication since the Solu-Medrol makes you sick after each administration."

"Okay, thank you."

"How are you feeling?" he asked.

"I feel okay. I did eat. My husband brought me food from McDonald's. He has been giving me Sprite to ease my stomach."

"That's good. I am administering the nausea medication now."

I could feel when the medication was going into my veins. It was a warm sensation.

"I am done administering the nausea medication and now I am administering the Solu-Medrol," the doctor explained.

When I felt the Solu-Medrol entering my veins, it was a different kind of warm sensation. The feeling of that medication made me alert. It was like I could see clearly. My body became numb with no feeling of any pain. It was a scary feeling, yet a great feeling because I was no longer in pain.

"I am done administering your medication. How do you feel?"

"Numb, no pain and sleepy," I answered.

"But you are not nauseous or feeling sick to your stomach?"

"No, I am not."

"I am going to leave now," he told me. "I will see you later this morning, since it is another day. I will be giving you the last dose of the Solu-Medrol and hopefully by that time we will have all the lab results back with the cause of the pain. Most likely I will be discharging you with a referral to a specialist."

"Sounds good," I responded.

"She is on her way to sleep," my husband pointed out. "Thanks for everything."

"No problem!" the doctor smiled. "That's why I am here."

I fell asleep with the doctor still in the room talking to my husband.

I woke up with the urge to go to the bathroom. I looked over at my husband and he was out, sound asleep. I called his name as quietly I could but loud enough to wake him. I didn't want to be too loud to scare him out of his sleep. You see, ever since I have been in pain and couldn't sleep, he was always alert. I woke him up to escort me to the bathroom and as always, he jumped up, thinking something was wrong.

"What's wrong? Are you in pain? Are you okay?"

"I am okay, I just need to go to the bathroom."

"Okay," he said, rubbing his eyes. "I am getting up."

As always, he helped me out of the bed, escorted me to and from the bathroom and back to the bed. Once I was back in bed, it didn't take me long to go to sleep. I was out.

I woke up again with the urge to use the bathroom. I knew it was the fluid from the IV bag that had me going. I looked over at my husband and he was already awake, watching television.

"Good morning."

"Good morning. How are you feeling?"

"I need to go to the bathroom."

He immediately got up and escorted me to the bathroom and back into the bed.

"Are you feeling any pain?" he asked.

I closed my eyes briefly. "Just a little, but not much. I know it's there."

"It's probably because it is wearing off and it's almost time for your last dose," said my husband. "I sure hope this doctor has found out what's going on with you so you don't have to suffer no more."

"I hope so, too."

There was a knock on the door, and then it opened. It was a male bringing my breakfast in. "Good morning, I have your breakfast. Would you like for me to bring the cart over to you?"

"Good morning," I answered. "No, thank you. I'll get it later."

"Okay, whenever you are done, just put it to the side and someone will be back later to pick it up."

"Okay, no problem and thank you."

After he left, I asked my husband to help me to the bathroom. This time I wanted to wash my face and brush my teeth. Once I was finished, he escorted me back to the bed. He then went back into the bathroom and washed his face and brushed his teeth.

There was a knock on the door and it slowly opened. It was my doctor. "Good morning, and how did you sleep?"

"Good morning," I responded. "I slept well. The only time I woke up was when I had the urge to go to the bathroom."

"It's your fluids from your IV bag."

"That's what I told my husband."

My husband entered the room from the bathroom, locking the door behind him.

"Good morning," he addressed the doctor.

"Good morning. I am here to administer her last dose of the Solu-Medrol and the nausea medication to keep her from getting sick. I also have the results back from all your labs. First let me administer the medications."

After the doctor finish administering both medications, he began with my lab results.

"All of your labs came back normal accept for your inflammation." he explained. "The labs I ran for lupus early detection also came back normal. Now that doesn't mean you do not have lupus. I am only allowed to do so much here in the ER."

"So, you are telling me I have to follow up with a rheumatologist for further testing"? I asked.

"Yes, that's exactly what I am saying. I am going to release you today with a prescription for prednisone until you make an appointment with the rheumatologist I suggest you see. He is one of the best rheumatologists here in Houston and Sugarland."

"What is the prednisone going to do?" my husband asked. "Is that safe for her to take without any problems?"

"I am just going to give her enough until she sees the rheumatologist. I will include directions on how to take it. She will be taking a mild dosage which will slowly increase to a semi-high dosage. Once she sees him, he will advise her on how to wean off it if he wants her to stop taking it."

"Okay, I just want to be sure about that particular medication," said my husband. "I do know that is a steroid."

"Yes, it is," the doctor confirmed. "But that is the only thing I can send her home with to give her some relief until she sees the rheumatologist."

"I sure hope this doctor can diagnose me," I added. "I am dreading leaving here knowing that awful pain will return."

"It shouldn't be as bad as it was when you first got here. The prednisone should give you some relief just like the Solu-Medrol did."

"What about work?" my husband asked. "Does she need to stay off until she sees the rheumatologist?"

"It's up to her," the doctor nodded in my direction. "If for some reason she starts experiencing uncontrollable pain, she shouldn't go to work."

"Okay, I will keep a close eye on her," my husband promised.

The doctor continued. "I am sorry I couldn't make a diagnosis. I am going to go and start your discharge paperwork. I will be including the referral to the rheumatologist with all of his office information, a list of your medication you are currently taking, including what we were giving you here in the hospital, a copy of your complete records, and my contact information just in case you or the rheumatologist need to contact me. It has been a pleasure treating you. I really pray you can be diagnosed immediately so you won't be in all of that pain."

"Thank you for all of your help," my husband told him. "Most of all, thank you for taking the time to listen to us and making an effort to find out her primary diagnosis."

"Yes, thank you for all of your help," I added.

"You two are very welcome. I will be sending the nurse back to discharge you. Now before I leave, are there any questions or concerns either of you may have?"

We both responded in the negative.

"Okay, good luck to the two of you." The doctor left the room.

My husband started gathering all of our things and packed them up. We sat there patiently, ready to go. I couldn't wait to get home to take a shower. The hospital bathroom only included a toilet and a sink. My husband called our sons, informing them that we would be home shortly. He then took all of our belongings to the car so that all he had to do was help me to the car without carrying all of those extra bags.

Finally, after 6:00 pm, the nurse came in with my discharge papers. She went over the discharge dos and don'ts with us, handed my husband my copies of the discharge papers with the prescriptions, and I signed the discharge forms. She wished us well and we left.

Chapter 11

The walk from the room to the car seemed like it took us forever to get there. I tried thinking positive thoughts about the next steps, seeing the rheumatologist and being diagnosed with my primary diagnosis and learning what was causing the swelling from the inflammation, the weight gain, the butterfly rash on my face, the discolored speckled pattern on both of my legs, and of course, the high temperature.

Once we were home, my husband helped me out of the car and through the front door. I greeted and kissed our two sons and greeted our Bichon, Trixter. I got in the shower, and from there, into our bed. We have a king size sleigh bed so my husband went into the garage and got our step stool to help me up and into the bed. He turned on the television, put a couple of my favorite DVDs in, and gave me the remote, making sure I was comfortable. He kissed me and off to the pharmacy he went.

The only way I was comfortable was lying on my back with two pillows under both of my knees. When my husband returned with the medications, I started the prednisone as directed. Since it was Thanksgiving, I didn't have to work and I had to wait until Monday to make my new patient appointment with the rheumatologist. During this time, I received phones calls and texts from family and friends. I also received a call from one of my cousins telling me that my great aunt had passed. I had to explain to her that I had just gotten out of the hospital and I wouldn't be able to make it to her funeral. She understood and wished me well.

On the following Monday, I called the rheumatologist's office from work. I was given an appointment within two weeks from the date I called. The doctor I worked for made it possible for me to change my arrival and departure times for work. Instead of going in from 8:30 am - 5:30 pm, I was now going in from 9:00 am or 10:00 am until 3:00 pm. He changed it because of the distance I had to drive and the traffic. It put a strain on my legs to drive and caused me to experience more pain. I did not want to stop working because, to me, it was like giving up. I have always been an energetic person with a personality to die for. I have always put people in my shoes before judging them. I would give my last effort to a person in need.

After just a few days of being on the medication, I started catching a cold. I was coughing, running a high temperature, and had a sore throat and stopped-up nose. My fever had gotten so out of control, I ended up at the ER. After having a throat swab and blood drawn, the results came back positive for the flu. On top of everything else that was going on with my health, I had the flu. It seemed as if I wasn't winning any kind of way.

On top of everything else that was going on with me, I was off of work, at home, in the bed with the flu. During that time, I received a call from the rheumatologist's office with an earlier appointment. I explained to the girl on the phone that I was home with the flu, but it was almost gone. She went ahead and scheduled me to come in that Monday, which was in three days. I scheduled it and made sure I had the correct address.

(Nowadays, the new patient forms are online on the doctor's office website. It really helps to get the forms early and fill them out before the appointment. The new patient forms are always a brain twister. Most likely, the questions are about family health history. The questions really put your brain to work.)

My husband was in the room with me when I received the phone call. He was happy the rheumatologist appointment was just a couple of days away. He then went into the living room and explained the update to our sons. Everything that was going on with me and my health was always communicated to our sons and the rest of our family and close friends so they could stay informed.

On Monday, I left an hour early from work to get to my appointment to see the rheumatologist. For one, I knew the area where it was, but I didn't know exactly where it was. I called my husband to inform him I was leaving work. The walk from the office building to the car was excruciating. The pain was getting worse the further I walked. I was constantly hurting, but it didn't hurt as much when I was sitting down. It was excruciating when I stood up on my legs and when I walked. It seemed as if someone was drilling into my bones. The feeling was also like a bad toothache -- you know that dull, aching, throbbing annoying pain. I wanted so badly to just dig into my bones and press down really hard. But of course, I knew better. I didn't do it.

Once I got to my car, I had to turn sideways to sit, and the tears flowed down my face in agony. Next, I lifted my right leg and gently swung it into the car. Finally, I did the left leg the same way. It took a lot out of me to get situated and comfortable in the car. The next step was pressing on the gas and brakes when needed. All the way to the rheumatologist's office, I cried from the pain.

When I got there, I called my husband to let him know I made it. He could tell by my voice I had been crying. He comforted me with soothing words. I ended the call and dreaded what was next. I really didn't look forward to the walk from the car to the building. Not only that, there was construction going on and it included a detour. It took me at least fifteen minutes to walk from my car to the office door. By the time I got to the floor the office was on, I looked at my watch to see how much time I had before my appointment. I still had twenty minutes to spare. I went into the ladies' room, hoping I was the only one in there because I just needed to cry from all of the pain I was in.

I finally made it to the rheumatologist's office. I signed in, gave the girl at the window my new patient's forms, she collected my payment, and I sat down. Within five minutes I was called to the back to the exam room. The medical assistant checked my vitals, asked necessary questions about my chief complaint, current medications, discontinued medications, and if I had any previous medical records. I handed her the medical records from my primary care doctors and the emergency records, including all of the scans. She was very impressed and amazed that I came prepared until she realized I worked for a neurologist/psychiatrist. (I try not to let medical office staff know where I work just to see how professional they are. Once they find out you work in the medical field, they always try to be on their best behavior.) Shortly after she exited the room, the rheumatologist came in.

"Good afternoon," he greeted me. "I looked over your medical records and the forms you filled out for today's appointment. You have been experiencing this pain off and on for quite some time now. Can you please explain to me what has been going on?"

Once again, I explained my history. "Back in 2015, I was admitted into the hospital for excruciating pain in my lower back and both legs to the end of my knees, elevated blood pressure, and increased temperature. The admitting doctor tried decreasing the pain by giving me morphine, but it didn't work. He couldn't find the reason for the pain, elevated blood pressure, and high temperature so he admitted me to further test me. They ran numerous scans on me, Dopplers, X-rays, and took a lot of blood, but nothing came back to explain why I was in so much pain. I was discharged without a primary diagnosis and with pain medication. I followed up with one of the neurologists I worked for regarding the pain. He thought it was neurological because of the severe pain in my legs. He tested me by doing an EMG on both legs. Nothing, my test was normal. After days, nights, weeks, and months went by, the pain disappeared until this year."

"So, you are telling me you haven't experienced the pain again until now?" the rheumatologist asked.

"Yes."

"How many doctors have you seen since the pain reoccurred?" he asked.

I began listing all my doctors. "My primary care doctor, her colleague because she was on vacation, two different ER doctors because I went twice to the hospital my primary doctor is affiliated with, the neurologist I used to work for, the ER doctors when I was admitted, and another one when I had the flu."

"I see you are taking prednisone," he said. "I am assuming it is for the pain."

"Yes."

"Is it helping?"

"Yes, but not as much as the Solu-Medrol did when I was in the hospital."

The rheumatologist looked at me. "I am going to start weaning you off because it's not good to be on it for a long period of time. Is this the first time you have taken the prednisone?"

"Yes, it is."

"Do you know your pharmacy number so I can send over a prescription electronically?"

I took my phone out of my purse and verbally gave him the number for the pharmacy close to my house.

"Now, I would like you to do a few things for me. I want to check your mobility."

"Sure."

The rheumatologist asked me to stand, walk to the door, step up on the stepstool for getting on the examining bed, bend and touch my toes, and raise my hands above my head. As I was doing those things, he asked me to rate my pain on a scale of 1 to 10, with 10 being severe.

"I am going to review all of your medical records. I have sent over your prescription to the pharmacy. I do know that there is something causing the pain, inflammation, and high temperatures. I can't say whether or not it is related to my specialty until I test you further. I want to see you back in a week to follow up after I review your records. Do you have any questions for me?"

"My only question is what I have been asking all of the other treating doctors. What is causing all of this pain?"

"I really don't know," he admitted, "but I am not going to give up until I find out. Can you please give me a chance?"

"Yes, what do I have to lose? I can only take it one day at a time until I find out the primary diagnosis."

The rheumatologist exited the room. Within minutes after he left, the medical assistant came in the room and gave me the instructions on how to wean off the prednisone. She then asked me to follow her to her desk to make my follow-up appointment. It took me a few minutes to get out of the chair because of the pain. Once we got to her desk, she made my one-week follow-up appointment. She gave me my appointment card and I left.

It seemed like it took forever to walk to my car. Whatever was going on with me was causing me to be immobile. Once I made it to my car and got comfortable, I called my husband to let him know I was on my way home. I couldn't wait to get home, into the shower, and in my bed. I left the doctor's office before the 5:00 pm rush hour traffic started. Pushing on the brakes and the accelerator made it harder on my legs. I couldn't wait to get home.

My husband was standing in front of the garage when I pulled up in the driveway. He instructed me to stop and not pull into the garage. I parked the car and got out. He helped me in the house. I spoke to our sons, greeted our puppy, got in the shower, and into the bed. My sons came in, asking questions about my appointment. I explained to them and my husband how everything went, including the painful, awful drive and walk to the rheumatologist's office. They all stood at the foot of my bed with heartbreaking and concerned looks on their faces. I knew my family hated that I was in so much pain and going through what I was going through. That's why I tried to stay strong. Not only for me but for my family as well. I knew that if I showed them any signs of breaking to the point of giving up, they would too.

Chapter 12

The week prior to my follow-up appointment, I started weaning off the prednisone. In the beginning, I was feeling fine. But by the time I went to see my rheumatologist, I could feel the pain slowly creeping back to where it was before. During my second appointment, my doctor suggested I see a neurologist and be tested for a neurological diagnosis. He then gave me several requisitions for bloodwork.

I explained to him that I wanted to see the doctor I used to work for. With his specialty and qualifications, he was an expert at what he did. He specialized in rare diseases, and if anyone could find out what was wrong with me, he could. Not only did I know him from working for him, I also trusted him.

My rheumatologist agreed with me seeing him. He had no problems with that. He then strongly suggested that I get completely off the prednisone.

I explained to him that I was following the instructions his medical assistant gave me. I also explained that the pain was slowly coming back as before.

After finishing up with my rheumatologist, I went to see his medical assistant. She asked me to call and make a follow-up appointment to see him after I saw the neurologist. She told me because it was late, the lab office was now closed and I would have to come back the next day to do the bloodwork. She also suggested that if I had any problems or concerns before coming back to see him, to just call the office and someone could help me. I thanked her and left.

As always, I called my husband and informed him on everything that was going on with me. And yet again, I dreaded the drive home. But I looked forward to getting in the shower and then into my bed.

The next day, I called the doctor I worked for and told him I needed a day off because I had to go get some tests done. He was okay with it.

My husband drove me to do my bloodwork. Once we got to the building, he tried parking as close as he could. As he escorted me to the lab office, he noticed my walking was slower than before. "Baby, are you alright? Do you want to sit?"

"No, I just want to get this over with and be back in my bed," I said.

"Are you sure? That lab office will be there."

"I am sure."

I really wished I had listened to my husband and sat down. The pain from my lower back to my knees was excruciating. It seemed as if I was carrying a ton. We finally made it to the door of the lab office. I was hoping and praying there weren't a lot of people in there. When we walked in, there were only four people sitting in the waiting area. I was happy.

My husband checked me in, gave the receptionist my lab orders and helped me sit next to the door that led to where they took your blood. After sitting for almost 30 minutes, I was called to the back. The young lady that called me looked at my requisition and explained to me that I was to come straight to the back because my doctor, the rheumatologist, checked off 'stat/patient is at high risk/can't sit long'. She was upset because the people who checked me in when we first got here were supposed to send me straight to the back.

"It's okay," I told her. "I just need to go to the ladies' room. Do you need to collect a urine sample from me before I go?"

"No, I just need blood from you. You can go and I will be right here waiting for you. There's an emergency cord on the wall if you need help."

I slowly walked to the bathroom. When I came out, the lab technician was waiting on me. She had everything prepared for me when I sat in the chair. She put on a pair of gloves, prepped my inner arm with an alcohol wipe, and inserted a butterfly needle in my vein. She then inserted tube after tube until she filled all the empty tubes she had laying on the tray next to me. Once she was done, she applied a cotton ball and then a nonstick Band-Aid on my inner arm. She helped me out of the chair and escorted me back to the waiting room where my husband was. She explained to us that my doctor would receive the results in a few days.

My husband took my arm and escorted me back to our car. I so dreaded the walk to the car. For once, I wished I had a wheelchair to use for these long walks. I knew my husband could see in my face that I was in pain. I just didn't want to feel hopeless. I never had to depend on anyone and I wasn't about to start now.

Once we were back home, I called the neurologist's office and made a new appointment. Because I used to work for the neurologist I was seeing, the scheduler who made my appointment already knew me. She was there before I had started working there and she was still there after I left. Instead of giving me the next available appointment, she asked me when I wanted to come in.

"Monday?" I suggested.

"What time?"

"I want to be his first patient," I told her. "What about 8:30 am? Is that available?"

"For you, yes."

"Okay, I will be there. Can I print out the new patient forms online or do I need to provide you with my fax number to fax them to me?"

"Yes," she said, "you can print the forms out online and bring them in with you. Let me know when you get here so I can come out to the waiting room and see you."

"Okay, will do."

"Alrighty, I will see you soon. Have a great day."

We said our goodbyes and ended the call.

I lay down in my bed with two pillows under my knees, trying to get comfortable. Our bedroom, our bed, and our television were now my new best friends. The only thing that could ease the pain some was being off of my feet, in my bed, on my back with two pillows under my knees. I lay in my bed just trying to keep a clear head and think positive thoughts. I did not want to think the worst. I was always reminded not to give up by my family and closest friends. My sisters called me on a daily basis, checking on me for updates on my health. They wanted to know what the doctors said, the doctors' specialties, what test I had to do, the name of the blood test, my next appointment dates and times, and how long it would take to get the results back from the tests. They were happy I was seeing the neurologist I used to work for. They knew he was a great doctor because I used to brag about him while working for him. He is really good at what he does.

After my third week of weaning off the prednisone, I suddenly was hit by a different type of pain. I never felt this pain before. The pain generated from my hips to the inner thigh, down to the top of my knee. I screamed out so loud my husband and sons came running in.

"Are you alright? What's wrong, baby?"

"The pain, the pain!" I exclaimed.

"Where are you hurting?"

I was rocking my hips from left to right, left to right. I shouted, "My hip, my right hip! It feels like someone is breaking my bones in my hip!"

"What can I do?" my husband asked. "What do you need?"

"I don't know what to do!" I moaned.

"Do you want the heating pad?"

"Yes, please!"

"Okay, let me go get an extension cord!" My husband hurried out of the room.

Both of our sons stood there with hurt in their eyes. I could see they were hurting for me. I tried assuring them that I would be just fine. But this time, they both were like, "Mom, you are not going to be without pain until they find out was causing all of it."

My husband came back in our bedroom, plugged the heating pad into the extension cord and into the wall. He asked me where I hurt; I showed him and he put the heating pad where the pain was and turned the heating pad on.

"Is the heating pad giving you some relief?" he asked.

"No, not really."

"What about an ice pack? Do you think that will help?"

"I am not sure, but we can try."

"I'll go get it, Dad," my oldest son offered.

Our son came back with the ice pack. My husband removed the heating pad and placed the ice pack on my hip. I ignored the cold sensation from the ice pack, just hoping it would help ease the pain.

"You know, you weren't in this much pain when you were taking the prednisone the way the emergency doctor prescribed it," my husband remarked. "You didn't start experiencing this much pain until the rheumatologist started weaning you off. You should give them a call and explain to them what is going on."

I held out my hand. "Give me the phone so I can call them."

Our youngest son grabbed the phone and handed it to me. I looked up the rheumatologist's number and called the office.

The receptionist answered, "Good afternoon, how may I help you?"

"Good afternoon, I need to talk to the medical assistant."

The line was silent for a moment, then the medical assistant answered, "Good afternoon, how may I help you?"

I identified myself and told her I was experiencing a lot of pain. "It has come back like before."

"When did the pain come back?"

"Today, right before I called you."

"Did you do anything to aggravate it?" she asked.

"No, it started after I followed the rheumatologist's weaning-off instructions. I am now going on the last week and I am in a lot of pain."

"I am going to talk to the rheumatologist and call you back. Is this a good number to call you back at?"

She confirmed my home phone number with me and we hung up.

"What did they say?" asked my husband.

"His medical assistant said she would talk to the doctor and call me back."

"Do you think she will call you back right away?"

"I am new to that office so I really don't know. If she doesn't call me back in 30 minutes, I will be calling her back."

After a few minutes, the phone rang. It was the medical assistant from my rheumatologist's office.

"The doctor just called in something for you for pain to your local pharmacy that is on file," she told me.

"Okay, thank you."

"You are welcome. I hope you feel better. Have a nice day."

We hung up. I told my husband that the doctor called me in something for the pain. He immediately put on his shoes, brushed his hair, grabbed the car keys and left. I lay in the bed, rocking from side to side, patiently waiting for him to get back with the pain medication. My sons stayed in the room with me until he returned.

When my husband got back, he set the medication on my night stand next to me, then made me a sandwich so I could take the medication. I ate the sandwich, took the medication, and waited patiently for the pain to ease up. Just a few more days before I could see the neurologist.

Chapter 13

Every day was a challenge. I never could predict what my mornings, afternoons, or nights were going to be like. I just took it one day at a time.

In January 2014, I went online and completed the necessary forms for the Obamacare healthcare insurance. They asked so many questions and asked for information on everyone in the house. I made sure I completed everything correctly on the forms. After I completed the forms, I received an answer right away. We were approved through the healthcare market for health insurance at an affordable monthly rate. It prompted me to pick an insurance plan. I looked over each plan one by one to make sure I picked a plan that all of my upcoming doctors accepted. From working in the medical field and verifying insurance benefits and eligibility as one of my job responsibilities, I knew which plan to get. I went to the insurance website, completed all of the necessary information, picked an insurance plan, and pressed Submit. Within seconds, the decision for the plan was granted. It gave me information about the cost per month, how to submit payment, and a booklet about the plan. I was one happy person.

I explained the insurance information to my husband and he was grateful that I now had insurance coverage for doctors' visits, lab work, images, and medications. Of course, in case I would need hospital or surgery coverage, I had that, too.

With my insurance coverage, in order for me to see a specialist (neurologist, rheumatologist, etc.) I had to get a referral from my primary care physician. I called my physician and made an appointment for the very next day. Before I hung up, I gave the medical assistant my new insurance identification number, group number, and the phone number to call and verify benefits and eligibility.

On the morning of my appointment at my primary care physician's office, my husband signed me in and gave the front desk receptionist my insurance card to copy. She handed him some forms to fill out because it had been more than six months since the last time I saw her. After my husband filled out the forms, we sat there for at least 45 minutes before being called to the back. Once we got to the back, the medical assistant took my vitals. She was worried about my high blood pressure. She also recorded my weight and noticed an increase in the weight from the last time I was there. She told me she would be right back with the doctor.

"Hello there!" she greeted me. "How are you and what is going on with you? I have never seen you like this. Please explain."

"I really don't know. I have been to see several doctors, been to the ER several times and admitted into the hospital. It is a possibility it could be lupus, but they don't know."

"I can tell you are in a lot of pain," she commented. "You have also picked up weight, but I am sure it is from the inflammation."

"Yes, I was told I have a lot of inflammation. I also have discoloration in both legs and I am getting a butterfly rash on my upper cheeks."

"I want to take a look. I am going to give you a gown; just put on the gown and only remove your pants. I am going to step out of the room and I will be right back."

I did as my doctor asked and she was back within minutes. She took a look at both of my legs. She put on gloves and touched them. "It feels like both of your legs have a high temperature, but that is the inflammation that's causing them to be inflamed."

"Yes," I agreed, "that is what I was told."

"I want to get an EKG (an electrocardiogram, a test that checks for problems with the electrical activity of the heart), some urine and blood."

"Okay, no problem."

When the EKG was done and I had given them the requested samples, my husband and I left and went home.

Every day was such a challenge for me. The pain in my legs was so severe, I really didn't know how I was able to go on every day. I just prayed and prayed and prayed for this to be over really soon.

The day had come for my new patient appointment with the neurologist. My husband let me out at the front so I didn't have to walk far. Of course, as always, it seemed like forever to get to my destination. I entered the neurologist's office and said hello to everyone that was working in the front. I knew several of them. They came out and hugged me. I signed in, gave them my new patient forms and my driver's license, and sat down. Shortly after I sat down, my husband came in and sat next to me. A moment later, the supervisor came out, hugged me and asked me what was going on with me. My husband and I explained everything to her. She could remember back in 2005 when I was admitted with the same symptoms. She informed me that she would talk to the neurologist to give me a discount because I was a self-paying patient. In other words, I wouldn't have insurance until the beginning of February. She hugged me again and told me she would keep me in her prayers.

I was just chitchatting with my husband when I was called to the back. I followed the medical assistant to the patient exam room. On the way to the back, I was greeted by everybody I knew from when I worked there. Once we got to the room, the medical assistant asked me to have a seat.

"Everyone here seems to know you," she commented. "I am going to take your vitals."

"Yes, I used to work here."

She took my blood pressure, my pulse, respiration, and temperature. As always, everything was elevated. "Are these all the medications you are currently on?"

"Yes."

"I am done. The doctor will be in with you shortly. It was nice meeting you."

"Okay, thank you. I am looking forward to seeing him."

The medical assistant left the room and the doctor came in.

"Well, looka here!" he said with a big smile. "It's been a while. When I saw you on the schedule, I was trying to figure out why you were coming in. Tell me what's going on with you."

"The pain that I had in 2005 is back. Remember, when I was working here, I was admitted into the hospital with severe pain in my lower back and both legs? After I was released you did an EMG on both of my legs. Well, guess what, it is back."

"Yes, I do recall," he said. "Back then when I did the EMGs, they were normal."

"Yes."

He looked at me closely. "You have a lot of inflammation on you. I can see it in your face and in your legs."

"Yes, every time I had lab work done, the inflammation test always came back positive," I told him.

"I see you have records from the same hospital twice, your primary care medical records, admission records, and the rheumatologist."

"Yes, the rheumatologist wants you to test me to make sure I do not have any neurological problems."

"I am sure it is not neurology-related but I will do an EMG on you."

"Okay, how soon do you want me to do it?"

He consulted my chart. "I see your insurance starts in a few days, so let's do it then. Why is your rheumatologist weaning you off the prednisone when you haven't been diagnosed? You haven't been on it long enough to cause any damage."

"I don't know," I answered. "I do know that when I was taking it the way the emergency doctor prescribed it, I wasn't experiencing a lot of pain. But when the rheumatologist starting weaning me off and I got close to completely off it, the pain came back."

"I want you to gradually go back up to taking it twice a day until we find out what is causing the pain. I am going to exam you now."

Once the neurologist examined my upper and lower extremities and reflexes, checked my eyes and my hearing, he was finished examining me. He sent over a few prescriptions electronically for the inflammation and for prednisone. When he was done, he walked me out to the nurses' station to check out. He had the medical assistant schedule the EMG for 8:30 am in two days. He hugged me and went in to see his next patient. The medical assistant gave me my appointment card, then I walked to the checkout desk and paid for the appointment with one of the girls I knew from when I worked there. We talked for a few minutes, she gave me my receipt, and I left with my husband. He went on ahead of me to go get the car so I didn't have to walk far.

The next few days were very challenging with the exhaustion from the pain. Regardless of what I did, I could not shake the pain. I am neither a whiner nor complainer, so I just tried tolerating it as much as I could. My husband and sons tried any and everything to make me comfortable. I was very appreciative and thankful for everything they were doing for me.

Finally, the day came for me to have the EMGs. I thought this day was never going to get here. I got up two hours early because it now took me an hour to get dressed. Before I got sick, I was dressed within 30 minutes. That included doing my hair and my makeup. Once I was dressed, my husband and I were out the door. From our house to my neurologist's office at 8:00 am would take at least an hour and a half to get there because of the rush hour traffic. With the pain I'd been experiencing, I'd rather not be in traffic sitting in that seat alone.

My husband dropped me off at the patient drop-off so I didn't have to walk far. I slowly walked into the building, got on the elevator, and went in my neurologist's office. I spoke to everyone, signed in, and sat down. Just when my husband was coming in the door, they called me to the back. To my surprise, it was one of the girls that had been there before I started working there and she was still here. She hugged me and said she was surprised to see me on the schedule. We chitchatted all the way to the testing room. She prepped me before the neurologist came in.

My neurologist came into the room and explained what he was getting ready to do. As he was doing the EMG on me, he predicted the test was going to be within normal limits. He said the only reason he was doing it was to clear me of the neurological diagnosis.

I did not disagree with him, not one bit. After all, he was the neurology specialist and he had many years to back him up.

It didn't take long for my neurologist to complete the EMG on both of my legs. He noticed the speckled patterns on both of my legs and said he had seen it before. He asked me to go ahead and get dressed and meet him at the nurses' station.

Once I was dressed, I had to ask my ex-coworker to help me put my shoes on and tie them for me. She helped me without hesitation. I hugged her and thanked her for helping me with my shoes. I explained to her that my husband was the one that helped me with my shoes and anything else I was limited to.

When I got to the nurses' station where my neurologist was standing, he gave me several lab requisitions to be tested for rare diseases. He also had the medical assistant schedule me an appointment in a week.

He explained to me that if anything came back abnormal before the follow-up, he would call me. He handed me the lab requisition and the appointment card, and I thanked him. I met my husband in the lobby and we left.

My husband and I took the elevator to the floor the lab office was on. Once we got to the receptionist's desk, my husband signed me in and we both sat down. Not long after we were seated, a lab technician called me back. She drew the necessary blood for the tubes she had beside me, then explained to me that my doctor would receive my final results within 72 hours. I thanked her and she escorted me to the waiting room where my husband was waiting.

When we got home, I took a shower to wash all of the gel off of my legs from the EMG, and I got in my bed. I was watching television when pain hit me so hard in both of my legs, I cried out in agony. My husband came running in the room from the living room.

"What's wrong?" he asked. "What happened? What did you do?"

"It hurts soo bad!" I cried.

"Do you want me to call the rheumatologist?"

"No, get my neurologist on the phone."

My husband grabbed the phone, but before he could dial the number, I asked him for the phone.

I dialed the number and the automatic recording came on. I pressed 0 for a live person. I was so happy the girl that answered the phone knew me from when I worked there. She could tell I was in some type of pain just by talking to me. I asked her to please transfer me to my neurologist.

"Hey, there!" he answered. "That was quick. What's wrong?"

I explained to him how the pain was a different kind of pain from all the previous ones. I told him that I couldn't take it anymore and that it had been going on too long and I still didn't have the answers.

"Where exactly do you hurt?"

"My lower back, my hips, my legs and my knees."

"What dosage of the prednisone are you taking? Are you still weaning off of it?"

"Yes, I am still weaning off."

"I want you to go back on them," he said. "I do not want you to wean off until I find out what is going on with you. Have you had an MRI of both of your legs, your lower back, your pelvis and your knees?"

"Yes, on everything except my pelvis."

"I am going to order an MRI on both of your legs, knees, your lower back and pelvis," he told me. "I am also going to order an X-ray on your pelvis and lower back. I am going to send the orders to the hospital so you can have them done. Give me an hour. I will have the medical assistant call you once the orders have been sent over. Don't forget to go back up on the prednisone so it can give you some relief."

"Okay, I will call the MRI facility in an hour. Thank you so much for all of your help. Oh, by the way, I am claustrophobic."

"No problem," he assured me. "I will have the medical assistant call something in for that. The directions will be on the bottle. I am going to get to the bottom of this. I want to get you back to your normal self. I can see you are in a lot of pain. I almost didn't recognize you when you came in on your first visit. Now make sure you call me if you need me."

"Okay, thanks again."

I explained to my husband and our sons what the neurologist told me.

They all were happy he was helping me. I was grateful for him.

I called the MRI facility to see if they had my orders from my neurologist. The receptionist asked for my date of birth and my doctor's name, and confirmed that she had received the orders. "Can you come in tomorrow morning?" she asked.

"Yes, I will be there."

"Okay, please be here 45 minutes before your scheduled appointment. Make sure you bring your identification. Do you need me to give you the address of where to come?"

"No, I know where you are located and I will bring my driver's license."

When I got off the phone, I explained to my husband and sons about the appointment for the scans. It looked as if things were falling into place. Hopefully, it wouldn't be long before I would be given a diagnosis for what was causing all of this pain.

Chapter 14

I called the pharmacy to see if anything had been called in from my neurologist's office. I was told that nothing had come through from him for me. I hung up with the pharmacy technician and called my neurologist's office back, but the office was closed. I left a message on the nurse's phone informing her that the doctor was going to send something over to my pharmacy to sedate me in order for me to have the scans. I left my name, date of birth, pharmacy number, and my phone number, then hung up.

The day was gone and night had come. Before I knew it, it was time to get up and get my ready for my tests. I called my pharmacy one last time before we left for my scans but I was told yet again that nothing had been called in. After I was dressed, I called my neurologist's office one last time to see if my prescription was sent to my pharmacy. The medical assistant checked the system but nothing was sent over. I left her a detailed message to give my neurologist regarding not having my sedation medication for the scans. Either way, I was going to have the scans. I wasn't going to let anything get in the way of me having them. For some strange reason, I felt like the scans he ordered would be what would finally find out why I had been in so much pain.

My husband and I left for the MRI facility. Once we got there, he let me out in front of the entrance door and I went in while he parked the car. I gave the receptionist my driver's license and she gave me forms to fill out. I took the forms and sat down. When my husband came in, I gave him the forms to fill out. I didn't fill them out myself because the severe lower back pain made my hands shake when I wrote. I am right-handed so my handwriting looked as if I wrote with my left hand. Once he was finished filling out the forms, he took them to the receptionist. Within minutes, I was called to the back to do my scans.

A radiology technician greeted me. "Good morning, I am here to take you to the back to do several scans on you. Have you had any scans before?"

"Yes, several," I answered.

"So, you know what to expect?"

"Yes," I told her, "but I am claustrophobic and my neurologist didn't send my prescription over so I could take it before my scans."

"It won't be so bad. I will help you through it."

"We shall see," I said, doubtfully.

We stopped in from of changing room. The radiology technician asked me to change into one of the hospital gowns. She said it opened in the back with two straps to tie them together. She told me when I was done to enter into the room to my left. When she walked out of the changing room, I changed into one of the gowns and tied it in the back like she instructed me to do, then walked into the room to the left.

The beast, I thought to myself. I really despise MRI machines. Just looking at it made me feel as if I was in a closed box and couldn't get out. The radiology technician saw me standing there, staring at it. She walked in and touched me on the shoulder. "It's going to be okay," she reassured me. "Before you know it, you will be done."

"I don't think so. I can already feel my throat closing up." I took a deep breath, trying to ignore the fatigue that was coming on.

"All you have to do once you are in the machine is close your eyes and think happy thoughts. Just go back to a time when you were happy and no one could steal your joy."

I took a deep breath. "Okay, sounds good. I can do this!"

"If for any reason, you just can't stay in the machine and complete the scans, I will stop and remove you."

I didn't argue with her. I told her to get this over with because it had to be done. She helped me up on the table connected to the big machine, positioned me properly, and walked behind me into the little control room. The lights went off where I was, and the table I was lying on started moving me into the big, round tube. After that, the pounding of the big machine began. I closed my eyes because I started panicking and thought about the birth of both of my sons. My heart stopped racing and before I knew it, the radiology technician told me it was over. I couldn't believe my ears. I was able to focus on something else that distracted me from being claustrophobic.

The radiology technician helped me off the cold, hard table onto the floor. I went into the patient dressing room where my clothes were and got dressed. Once I came out of the dressing room, the radiology technician escorted me back to the patient waiting room where my husband waited. She explained to me that my doctor would receive the images and reports electronically. I thanked her for all of her help and we left.

We weren't home a good hour when I received a call from my neurologist. I was afraid to answer the phone because I knew there was something abnormal with one of my scans.

I answered the phone. As I had feared, it was my neurologist's office.

"Can you come in tomorrow at 8:30 am?" the receptionist asked.

"There must be something wrong with my scans because you are asking me to come in before my scheduled follow-up appointment," I observed.

"You know I can't say. He asked me to call you right away and make sure you were here first thing tomorrow morning. Can you be here?"

"Yes, I will be there."

We said our goodbyes and hung up.

"What's wrong?" asked my husband.

"I was just asked to be at the neurologist's office at 8:30am!"

"There has to be something abnormal with one of your scans for her to call you in sooner before your scheduled appointment," he commented, echoing my thoughts.

"Yes, I am sure. I am just happy someone is finally getting to the bottom of all of this pain."

"That makes two of us."

I called my family and closest friends with an update on my status. They were concerned but happy we were finally getting somewhere.

The big question was, "WHAT COULD IT BE?"

Once our sons were home, we explained to them about the appointment I had for the following morning with my neurologist. They, of course, had concerned looks on their faces. I assured them that whatever it was, I was not going to give up. I was going to fight with everything in me and more. They both looked at me with some relief.

That night I had a hard time sleeping. I was excited and scared at the same time. I just couldn't help wonder what was wrong with me. I started having thoughts of some type of cancer, lupus, liver disease and other rare bone diseases. I tried thinking of happy thoughts but the fear of those diseases played over and over in my head. Before I knew it, it was time for me to get up and get ready for my appointment.

When my husband and I made it to my neurologist's office, I signed in but before I could sit down, I was called to the back. After the medical assistant took my vitals, she left and my neurologist came in.

"Good morning! How are you feeling?"

"Nervous about what you are about to tell me!" I admitted.

He looked at me and said, "You have avascular necrosis in both hips."

"Say that again!"

"You have avascular necrosis of both femoral heads in both hips. I know you are not familiar with the disease but that's why you are in so much pain. You have loss of blood to the bones in your hips which caused them to collapse. In other words, death of bone tissue due to lack of blood supply.

"Really, that explains the excruciating pain?"

"Yes! I can't believe you are still working and driving. Your bones and joints in both hips have collapsed."

"Oh, my God! What now?" My head was spinning.

"We need to get you to an orthopedic surgeon right away! But I want to refer you to someone that I know and trust."

"Surgery?"

"Yes! I am sorry to tell you, but both of your hips have to be replaced."

I was stunned. "I thought that was just for elderly people!"

"Not in your case," he explained. "You are in the last stage of this rare disease which now requires immediate surgery. I am going to have the medical assistant fax over your records to the orthopedic surgeon I suggest. But first, I need to make sure he accepts your insurance. I am going to need you to pick up all of your scans from the imaging facility and take them to your appointment. Come on out to the front so we can get you scheduled with the orthopedic surgeon ASAP. I am going to take you off of work and limit you on mobility. I still can't believe you have been mobile with your bones and joints like this. Oh, one more thing, go ahead and start weaning off the prednisone."

"Alright, if you say so."

"The orthopedic surgeon is going to suggest you be off of them before he performs surgery," he added.

Once we were at the nurses' station, my neurologist asked the medical assistant to print out all of my medical records, put them in an envelope, and give them to me to take to the orthopedic surgeon. He also asked her to give me the name and phone number of the orthopedic surgeon he wanted me to see.

When I met my husband out in the patient waiting room, I explained to him what the neurologist told me. He was surprised. It wasn't something we expected. We had never heard of such a diagnosis or illness before, but we were relieved because finally we knew the reason for the excruciating pain.

Once we were home, we explained everything to our sons. The looks on their faces were like a ton of bricks were lifted off of them.

Once I got settled in my bed, I called the orthopedic office that my neurologist referred me to. I explained to the receptionist that I was referred to this doctor by my neurologist for avascular necrosis of both hips. I asked her if the doctor accepted my insurance and sadly, he didn't. I told her how disappointed I was and said my goodbyes.

I asked my husband to bring me the laptop so I could look up orthopedic surgeons that were in the network with my insurance. I logged in, typed in 'orthopedic' and my zip code, and within seconds there was a list of in-network orthopedic surgeons. I googled them one by one until I found one with outstanding ratings and reviews. I wrote the information down, called the doctor's office, and was able to make an appointment for that same week. I was asked to bring previous medical records and all of my images.

When I hung up with the orthopedic office, I called the imaging facility and requested all of my images. I was told I could pick them up the next day. I explained to her I would pick them up the morning of my appointment at the orthopedic office. She said that would be fine and to just make sure I brought identification.

Next, I called my primary care office because now I needed a referral to see the orthopedic surgeon. I was given an appointment for the following morning. My primary care physician needed an update on my health status.

Bright and early the next morning, my husband and I went to see my primary doctor. We weren't sitting a good five minutes before we were called to the back. The medical assistant took my vitals and weight, and left the room since I was only there to give my primary care doctor an update on my health.

"Good morning!" my doctor greeted me. "I have received your records from your neurologist. I was surprised by what I saw as your diagnosis."

"Yes, I have been diagnosed with avascular necrosis of both hips. My femur bones have dislocated themselves from my pelvis. I have seen both a neurologist and a rheumatologist. My neurologist that I used to work for was the one who discovered the avascular necrosis and he has taken me off work. I am here because I have insurance that requires a referral for me to see the neurologist and the orthopedic surgeon for surgery."

"Oh, my good friend!" she exclaimed. "I am so sorry to hear you are going through all of this. I will provide you with whatever you need."

"She has been going round and round with doctors and hospitals," added my husband. "She was admitted into the hospital last year on her birthday with a possibility of having lupus. I am tired of seeing her in all of this pain. It took the doctor she used to work for to make a diagnosis."

My doctor shook her head. "I can only imagine. Avascular necrosis is a rare disease and it takes time to find it. It is a shame with all of the technology that is known, we can't pinpoint rare diseases until it is too late."

"You are right," said my husband.

"Friend, I am worried about your high blood pressure," said the doctor.

"Yes, I know. But we all know it is due to the excruciating pain and inflammation that's causing me to have the increase in weight gain."

"I am going to send the medical assistant in to get the names of the doctors you are needing the referrals for and have them fax it to them stat."

"Thank you," I told her.

She stood up. "Please keep me informed and up-to-date on your health status."

The doctor left the room and the medical assistant came back in. I gave her both my neurologist's and orthopedic surgeon's names, addresses, phone and fax numbers. She stated she was going to give the information to the referral receptionist and do it stat per the doctor. I thanked her, and then my husband and I got up and left.

On the morning of the appointment to see the orthopedic surgeon, we went by the imaging facility first so we could pick up all of my images. We left there and went to the orthopedic office. After my husband let me out at the front door and then met me in the orthopedic office, I signed in and gave the medical assistant my insurance card and identification. She handed me the new patient forms. Once I sat down, my husband took the forms from me and started filling them out. He had to check his phone to see what day it was; he looked at me and told me Happy Valentine's Day. We had been going and coming to the point where we didn't know what day it was.

When he was finished with the forms, I was called back by another medical assistant. We followed her to an exam room where she took my vitals and chief complaint. She helped me on the exam table and told us the doctor would be right in. Within seconds, the orthopedic doctor came in.

After we greeted each other, the doctor looked down at my chart.

"I see you were referred by your neurologist with a diagnosis of avascular necrosis of both hips. I have reviewed your records and imaging reports. I would like to check just a few things. Can you lie back for me?"

I did what he asked.

"I know you are going to want to hurt me for this, but I have to do it."

What happened next was not what I expected. The orthopedic doctor grabbed my right leg and swung it out toward the right. I almost died. The tears started flowing in full force down my face.

"Is she alright?" asked my worried husband.

"Yes, she is. I am sorry to tell you this, but she needs surgery ASAP. I need to get an X-ray of both hips and pelvis to confirm the severity of the avascular necrosis. I am going to send you downstairs to have them done and then I want you to come back up here. Once you have it done, the reports will come to me right away."

"No problem. Do we need to wait on the orders for the X-ray or are you going to send them over?" my husband asked.

"No, you don't need to wait on them. I will send them over stat."

"I so dread this walk downstairs," I said.

"I know you are in a lot of pain," the doctor told me. "I am going to make sure you are taken care of."

"I'll make sure she is alright," my husband added.

We left and went downstairs to the hospital imaging facility. Once we were there, my husband helped me sit down and then signed me in. He was given a form to fill out. After he completed the form and turned it in to the receptionist, I was called to the back. Once I was back there, I had to sign several documents in order to have the X-rays, and then I was asked to have a seat back in the lobby. Within minutes, I was called to the back to do the X-rays. Afterwards, I was escorted back to the lobby and we went back upstairs to the orthopedic office. Before we could sit down, we were called to the back.

"Just as I suspected!" the orthopedic doctor announced. "The AVN in both of your hips has caused both of your femur bones to collapse and they are severely brittle. You are in the last stages of the disease. Early detection is never caught on time. Unfortunately, the last stage is the stage when someone is diagnosed. During this stage, immediate surgery is required. What I am about to tell you is not good. You need to have surgery ASAP but you can't have them done at the same time. The second issue is, I don't do hip replacements. I only do minor surgeries."

"What?" my husband exclaimed. "Why did your staff schedule her when she explained to them the reason for coming here?"

"It is probably because my colleagues do hip replacements but none of them take your insurance."

"She has one of the best insurance plans!" my husband protested. "Her deductible is met at 100%, and with that being said, anything she has done is covered at 100% where she doesn't have to pay out of pocket."

"I really do understand and I am sorry," the doctor apologized. "So, it was just a waste of time coming here to see me. It's all about money."

My husband shook his head. "So, we are back to square one of finding an orthopedic surgeon that can treat her AVN and perform the hip replacements?"

"Well, I just need my medical records from you and my images back so I can take them to the orthopedic surgeon," I said.

"I am sorry for everything," the doctor repeated.

My husband and I made sure we had all of my images and the medical records we brought in, grabbed one of the orthopedic business cards and left. My husband went ahead of me so he could go and get the car and be waiting out in the front when I walked out of the building. We knew once we were home I had to look for an orthopedic surgeon that specialized in AVN.

Chapter 15

Once we got home, my husband made sure I was comfortable, gave me the laptop, and I got busy. I found one orthopedic surgeon who had a portfolio that caught my attention. I read all the reviews on him and from there I was satisfied. I went to his website, filled out the new patient questionnaire, and shortly afterwards, our home phone rang. When I looked at the caller ID, it was the orthopedic office for which I just completed the questionnaire. That was fast, I thought to myself.

I answered the phone. "Hello?"

"Hello, I am calling from the orthopedic office. We just received a questionnaire from you. When can you come in?"

"Before I schedule, I have a couple of questions," I said. "I know I had to enter my insurance and the reason I need to make an appointment. Does this specific doctor take my insurance and can he perform hip replacements on my hips?"

"Yes, ma'am, he accepts your insurance and he performs all orthopedic surgeries."

I breathed a sigh of relief. "Thank goodness! When can I come in?"

"We have something as early as Wednesday at 10:00 am. Can you come for that day and time?" she asked.

"Yes, I can."

"I see you have previous images and medical records," she said. "Can you please bring all that in to your appointment?"

"Sure, no problem. I see there are new patient forms online I can complete before I come in. Can I do so and will the doctor get it prior to my appointment?"

"Yes, please complete all of the new patient forms online."

"Thank you so much," I told her. "Have a great day."

"Same to you. See you Wednesday."

When morning came, we got up, dressed and out the door. We had to drive further than the previous doctors I'd seen. He was located in the medical center. When we got to the building where the orthopedic surgeon was, my husband let me out at the patient drop-off as usual. I waited for him to park the car, and then we went to the elevators that would take us to the doctor's office. He was located on the top floor and his office took over the entire floor. I was impressed. We walked up to the front desk, signed in, and was asked to give my identification and insurance card.

"Baby, go ahead and have a seat. I'll wait for your license and insurance card."

My husband watched me to make sure I was sitting down and then he turned his attention back to the receptionist. When she was finished making copies of my license and insurance card, she handed them to my husband. He then came and sat beside me. We sat there for 20 minutes before being called to the back. We followed the medical assistant into the exam room. We were amazed of everything that was in this office. The doctor had his own imaging room for MRIs, X-rays, etc. The medical assistant took my vitals and a brief history of my chief complaint, then told us the doctor would be in shortly.

As we sat there in the exam room, we could see the entire downtown of Houston. My husband took several pictures over the city. The sight was amazing.

The door slowly opened, and the orthopedic surgeon came in, a nurse following behind him.

"Hello!" he said. "How are you this morning?"

"I wish I could tell you I am doing fine, but that would be a lie," I answered.

"I see you have been diagnosed with avascular necrosis in both hips."

"Unfortunately, yes."

"You are only 39 years old, right?" asked the doctor.

"Yes, that is correct."

"I am reading the forms you filled out prior to coming in. Now you stated you were not involved in a car accident nor a bad fall, right?"

"That is correct," I repeated.

"You have never used steroids or prednisone until recently, right?"

"That is also correct."

"You stated you had two natural, normal births without any complications, right?"

"That is also correct."

"I am going to need you to lie back for me to check your hips, both legs and knees. I promise you, I won't hurt you."

I lay back as requested. The doctor was very gentle as he examined my hips, both legs and knees. He then helped me up.

"I see you have brought some films with you. I will need to take a look at them and I'll be right back. But in the meantime, this is my nurse. She will be asking you several questions. We are going to take care of you." He smiled reassuringly.

I thanked him and he left the room with all of my images.

His nurse came over to me. "I am looking at the forms you completed prior to this appointment. You have completed everything on here. Now, I see you have seen a neurologist, rheumatologist, orthopedic doctor, your primary care physician, ER, and you have been admitted into the hospital. I am going to get you a couple of medical releases so we can get your records."

"I brought them all with me," I told her. "My husband has them."

"Here you go," he handed my records over to her. "There are a lot of them."

"I see! She came prepared." The nurse looked impressed.

"I have worked in the medical field for a total of 13 years," I explained. "I know previous medical records are always requested. That way the doctor won't repeat any test."

"You are the only one that came prepared," she said.

The door opened and the doctor came in.

"You are in the last stage of avascular necrosis, which is also called osteonecrosis," he told me. "Your joints have collapsed in both hips which need total hip replacements immediately. I can only do one at a time. Tell me something, which hip is the worst?"

"My right hip," I answered.

"Yes, I thought so. I saw it on the images. I am going to have my nurse get you set up for your first hip replacement. She will be giving you something to do before I can perform the hip replacement."

"You are talking about a medical clearance?" I asked.

"You are one smart cookie," remarked the doctor. "Yes, I will need a medical clearance. I see you were on prednisone; how long have you been off of it?"

"Two weeks."

"Okay, that's good to know. Are you or have you been taking any aspirin?"

"No," I said.

"After the first hip replacement, I want to do the left hip replacement three to six months after the right hip. Once your hips are replaced, you will no longer feel the pain anymore. You will feel some discomfort, but not like what you are experiencing now."

"That's good to know."

"I am going to let my nurse give you everything you will need to clear you for your first surgery. My first day available will be in two weeks. If you can provide me with everything I need to clear you, I will see you then."

I nodded. "Okay, we will get on it right away."

"Here is a list of things we will need before we can put you on the schedule for the surgery," the nurse said, handing me a sheet of paper. "Once you have clearance, please ask the doctor to fax over the results ASAP."

"Okay, will do," I said. "Is there anything else we need to do before we leave?"

"No, that will be all," answered the nurse.

The orthopedic doctor and the nurse left the room, and we weren't far behind them. As we were walking towards the front, the nurse gave my husband her personal business card. She asked him to call her with any questions or concerns he may have. He took the card, thanked her, and we left.

My husband went ahead of me to get the car. Once he pulled up in front of the patient's pick-up/drop-off, I got in the car slowly and very carefully. The pain just seemed to be getting worse by the day.

On our way home, I called my primary care doctor's office and informed them I needed a referral to a cardiologist for clearance to have surgery. I also asked them to fax over my lab and urine results to the orthopedic doctor's nurse. I gave her the name and direct extension. I asked the person on the phone to repeat what I just told her because I didn't want any delays. When I was satisfied, I hung up and moved on to the next task.

After my primary care doctor's medical assistant called me to inform me it was okay to call the cardiologist's office to make my appointment, I thanked her and called right away. My scheduled appointment was for that Monday. I was so thankful that all the doctors I had to see got me in right away. I did not have to wait a month to be seen.

On Monday morning, my appointment at the cardiologist's office was quick. Due to the increase in my blood pressure, the cardiologist increased my blood pressure medication that I was currently on. He was concerned about my irregular heartbeat. I told him I was born with it and unfortunately, I was that one person that didn't outgrow it.

"You are so young to be having the health problems you are experiencing," he commented.

"I just want it all to go away," I told him, "especially the pain."

"I have received your records from your neurologist, primary care doctor, and the orthopedic doctor. I see you are scheduled to have your right hip replaced because of avascular necrosis. Do you have lupus that's causing the avascular necrosis in your hips?"

I shook my head. "No, it has not been diagnosed as the cause of the avascular necrosis."

"Have you had a long-term use of steroid for pain, asthma or any other autoimmune health issues?"

"No."

"I am going to go ahead and have my medical assistant send over the orders for the EKG that is requested by your orthopedic doctor," he said. "He needs it for clearance in order to perform the surgery."

"Yes, I am aware of it," I told him. "The sooner the better."

"I am going to send you next door to get your echocardiogram. I am going to have my medical assistant fax over the order along with your identification and insurance card. I am going to have her give you a copy of everything just in case they say they didn't get it. You do not need an appointment. The facility is affiliated with the hospital."

"Okay, I was going to ask for a copy of the orders because I know from experience, they tend to lose or say they didn't receive the orders."

"That's true," he admitted. "We get that all the time here. The fax machine will print out the confirmation it has been sent but yet they will say they didn't get it."

The cardiologist increased my blood pressure medication, sent a new prescription electronically to my pharmacy, gave me his business card, gave me the orders for the echocardiogram and told us he would see us after my surgery. He stated if the echocardiogram came back abnormal, he would see us before the surgery.

Once we got to the area for me to have the echocardiogram, my husband checked me in and the nightmare began. We were there for more than two hours and I still hadn't gotten the echocardiogram done. The two women at the desk didn't know what they were doing. They repeatedly told my husband they received the orders from the cardiologist office and someone would be calling me soon to have the echocardiogram done. After about 30 minutes, my husband went up to the receptionist's desk and asked them what was taking so long because I was having a hard time sitting in the chair. One of the ladies told my husband the orders hadn't come through from the cardiologist's office. My husband asked her why they didn't say that at first. He gave them the orders given to him by the cardiologist and told them to make a copy and give him back the original orders.

After phone calls to and from my cardiologist's office regarding the echocardiogram orders, and after sitting there for over two hours, we found out they didn't take my insurance and we would have to pay out of pocket for the echocardiogram. My husband had choice words with the ladies at the receptionist's desk. He asked for the orders, my identification, and insurance cards back and we left.

By the time we got home, it was after 4:00 pm. My husband explained everything to our sons, and then he helped me in and out of the shower, and into bed. Once I was comfortable in the bed, my husband brought me the laptop so I could look up an echocardiogram facility that was in-network and I wouldn't have to pay out of pocket. Just a co-payment and not the full price of the test.

I was in luck! I found a facility not far from our home. I called the facility and made an appointment. I gave the office my insurance information so they could verify it before my scheduled appointment. I didn't want any surprises.

On the day of my appointment for the echocardiogram, my husband and I left an hour early because I had to be there 30 minutes before my scheduled appointment to fill out forms. Once we got there, my husband checked me in, filled out the forms, paid my co-payment and sat down next to me.

We hadn't been sitting down long when I was called to the back. The radiologist technician asked me to remove my shirt and bra only and put on a gown. She said the gown opened in the front. Once I was ready, she helped me on the bed, cleaned my chest, and placed the electrodes. (An echocardiogram is an ultrasound test that uses sound waves to generate images of your heart. This allows the doctor to examine the shape, size, and movement of your heart, and assess how well it is working.) It took about 45 minutes to complete the test. I explained to the radiologist technician the report needed to be sent over to my doctor ASAP because my orthopedic doctor needed it before he could replace my hip. The radiologist technician told me the test was a stat and it was written on the sleeve of the echocardiogram. I thanked her for her services, got dressed, walked out to where my husband was, and we left.

It took me two days to get my results sent over to my orthopedic surgeon. I spent hours on the phone with the facility where I had my echocardiogram, my primary care doctor's office, the cardiologist's office and the orthopedic office. Once my orthopedic nurse received everything for my clearance, she scheduled my total right hip replacement for March 11, 2014 with the arrival time at the hospital for 5:30 am. I was one happy person. I could finally get rid of all this excruciating pain in my right hip.

On March 5, 2014, my husband and I attended a teaching class for the surgery. The nurse explained to us the dos and don'ts before and after my total hip replacement. We were given brochures that explained the surgery. The nurse explained how to use the walker and cane, and how to sit and get in and out of the bed.

After we left the teaching class, my husband and I went to the pre-admission department. There, I had to sign forms, choose the type of room I wanted after my surgery, and give more blood. Once I was done there, my husband and I went home.

I called my closest family and friends, informing them of my surgery. Everyone was happy that I had finally been diagnosed and now I was days away from being relieved of this excruciating pain.

The night before my surgery, I started getting scared. I didn't know if I would wake up after the surgery, I didn't know if I would die in the middle of the surgery. I just didn't know. I kept looking at the time in anticipation. When it was 4:00 am, I woke up my husband. He got up, took a shower, packed our bag for a three-night stay at the hospital, helped me get dressed, told our sons we were leaving and out the door we went.

Once we got to the hospital, my husband dropped me off at the patient drop-off door. Within minutes my husband came and sat next to me. As we sat there, people started coming in and filling up the waiting room. I was the youngest patient there.

After sitting for over 30 minutes, a middle-aged woman asked for the people that were there for surgery to please follow her. Everyone, including my husband and me, got up and followed her. When we got to the destination, we were called up one-by-one. When I was called, the nurse asked for my identification. She printed out several identification tags and put them on my wrist. She then had me fill out several forms. When I was finished, she asked me to have a seat back in the patient waiting area.

As I looked at my surroundings, I realized this was reality and not a dream. I was actually sitting here, waiting to be called to the back for major surgery. All of sudden, my throat felt dry. I began to get scared. My thoughts were interrupted by a nurse calling my name. She asked me to follow her. My husband came with me.

We were now in a different area of the hospital. The nurse asked me to take off all of my clothes and put the hospital gown on. She told me the gown should open in the back and then I could put the other gown on to cover the back. She then inserted a needle in my vein for my IV. The room was so cold, I asked for extra sheets to keep me warm. As I lay in the bed, my husband sat beside me in a recliner.

At 6:15 am, the nurse came in and told us it was time for me to go to the surgery area. My husband kissed me on my lips, and then the nurse wheeled me to the surgery area. I was surrounded by my orthopedic doctor, his nurse, and the anesthesiologist.

My orthopedic doctor greeted me and told me I was the first patient on his list to perform the hip replacement. He assured me that everything would be okay. He reminded me again that I was the youngest patient to have a hip replacement.

My nurse introduced me to the anesthesiologist. She said she was going to give me something to help me relax. She began injecting a clear fluid into my IV. She started to ask me a question but the next thing I knew, I was out.

Chapter 16

I woke up to the sound of my husband's voice. I slowly opened my eyes and followed his voice. He kissed me on the lips and told me, "Welcome back."

Shortly after, I heard a female voice on my left side. "I am your nurse while you are in the recovery room. I will be giving you something for the pain. Whenever you are in pain, push the red button and I will assist you."

"Okay," I mumbled. "Where is my husband? I don't see him."

"He is waiting in the patient lobby. Once your room is ready, someone will come get you, transport you to your room, and then your husband will join you."

"Okay, no problem. I am starting to feel pain."

"Let me check to see when you were last given something for the pain," the nurse said. "I will be right back."

I just lay there, waiting on the nurse to get back with my medication. Before she could come back to me, a porter showed up to transport me to my room. That was where I would be until I was discharged.

The nurse reappeared at my bedside. "I am going to give you something for the pain. It's been a while since you had something." She said to the porter, "Once I give her the pain medication, you can transport her to her room."

The nurse inserted the pain medication in my IV and wished me well on my recovery.

"Thank you so much," I told her.

The porter was unlocking my bed when I asked him to get my husband before pushing me to my room. He told me he would get him on the way to the room. When we got to my husband, he was excited to see me. He got up and followed us to the room.

Once we got to the room, the porter positioned my bed, locked it, and left. My husband pulled the curtains closed and turned on the television.

Taking my hand, he asked, "How are you feeling?"

"I feel sore, but I don't feel all of that excruciating pain that I was feeling before."

"That's good to know." He smiled at me. "One down and one more to go."

My husband was fixing my pillow when the nurse walked in. "How are you feeling?" she asked.

"I am okay," I told her.

"I know you haven't eaten anything. I am going to start you on something light and work your way up to solid foods. I don't want you to get sick to your stomach."

"Can you please remove the oxygen tubes from my nose?" I asked her. "They are driving me crazy. I am feeling claustrophobic with them in my nose."

"Oh, sure! You don't need that anymore."

The nurse removed the oxygen tubes, and then wrote on the board in my room the time she would be coming back to check on me. She also wrote the names of the medical staff assigned to me, including the doctor and the certified nursing assistant. She wrote the time when I was to receive my medications.

During my days in the hospital, I received calls from my sons, some family members and friends. My orthopedic doctor came to check on my status, and my orthopedic nurse changed my bandages (it hurt). They changed my pain medications and put me on blood thinners. I was given nausea medications when I felt sick and I had to wear support stockings on both legs.

I was assigned a physical therapist who taught me how to get in and out of the bed, how to sit, how to get up, how to get on and off the toilet, and how to walk up and down stairs. He also showed me how to do foot exercises in the bed to keep my blood flowing like it should. The support stockings and the foot exercises were to prevent blood clots. He also advised me that if I was sitting in a chair or on the couch, to use two pillows to raise me high off the chair or couch. He told me to make sure my legs weren't bent. They had to be out from the couch.

My orthopedic doctor advised me to walk laps inside the house several times a day, using my walker or cane. He told me if I was using my cane, to use my left hand to walk with the cane. He said the pressure should be used on the side opposite of the surgery site. He didn't want the pressure of walking to be on my right side where I had the hip replacement.

After three days in the hospital, I was finally going home. Before I left, I was educated on the dos and don'ts. My treating doctor sent all of my medications to my local pharmacy and the nurse made arrangements for my three-in-one toilet to be delivered to our home.

The nurse came in the room with the discharge forms for me to sign. After I signed the forms, the porter came in the room to take me downstairs. My husband grabbed all of our belongings, and left the room to go and get the car. He didn't want me to wait long so he went ahead of us.

After I was packed and ready to go, the porter took me downstairs and helped me into the car. My husband took his time driving home, trying to avoid every bump in the road. He didn't want to do anything that would cause me to have pain.

The first night I was home was a nightmare. I tried sleeping in our big king-size California sleigh bed, but nope, that didn't work. I was very uncomfortable. Nothing was going right. I asked my husband to make up the sofa in the living room for me to lie on. He grabbed four comforters out of the linen closet, folded each one lengthwise twice and placed them one by one on the couch. Then he grabbed a fitted sheet and covered the top comforter as if it was a mattress. He then grabbed another fitted sheet, placed it on top of the other fitted sheet and folded it back. My husband propped three pillows in front of the arm of the couch as if I would be sitting up in our bed.

I eased myself down to sit on the couch the way the physical therapist taught me. I then grabbed my right leg and carefully swung it onto the couch, and then did the same with the left one. I was now sitting up on the couch as if I was sitting up in our bed with my back against the headboard.

I still didn't feel comfortable. I asked my husband to bring me two pillows and prop them both underneath my knees. Finally, I got some relief.

As the days and nights went by, taking my scheduled medications, using an ice pack, sometimes a heating pad (not on the surgery site) and walking around the inside of the house, the discomfort from my right hip replacement slowly went away. The second week after my hip replacement, I went to see my orthopedic doctor for my two-week follow-up. He told me the right hip was looking good and I should be walking better in no time. I was happy to hear that. I no longer felt the excruciating pain like I did before. It was a dull aching pain I could tolerate.

Six weeks after my total right hip replacement, something unexpected happened. I was sitting up on the couch watching television, when all of sudden an excruciating pain hit me hard in my left hip. My husband was outside talking to my mother and my mother-in-law. I yelled for my oldest son. He came running into the living room to see what I needed.

As I tried to answer him, I couldn't talk for the tears that were flowing down my face. I screamed out several times in pain. This pain was different from all of the other times. My oldest son ran outside to get my husband. He came into the living room with our oldest son, our youngest son, my mother and his mother steps behind him.

"What's wrong?" he asked.

"The pain, the pain in my hip!" I cried.

"Your right hip?"

"No, my left hip! It's hurting really bad! I can't make it go away!"

"Should we take you to the ER?"

"No, I just need to ease the pain until tomorrow morning," I moaned. "I will call my orthopedic nurse first thing."

My husband glanced at his watch. "It is not yet time for your scheduled pain medication, but I don't think an hour will harm anything if you took it."

"Yes, please give me one!"

My husband grabbed my pain medication and a bottle of water. I took the pain medication hoping and praying it would give me some relief until the following morning. I sat on the couch, rocking back and forth, trying to ignore the pain, when the house phone rang. My husband grabbed the phone and answered it. It was my youngest sister calling to check on me.

"She is not having a good night," he told her. "She is having severe pain in her left hip. I don't think she is up to talking right now."

"No, it's okay," I said. "Maybe talking to her will distract me from focusing on the pain."

My husband gave me the phone. Everyone, my husband, our sons and my mother-in-law, stood there watching me while I talked to my sister. In the beginning of our conversation, I was crying, but as we kept talking and the medication kicked in, I eventually stopped crying and we hung up so I could try and get some sleep. Well, that didn't happen! I was wide awake. As the night went by, I watched television, searched the web on my cell phone, and listened to my husband and our puppy sleep.

At 9:00 am the next morning, I called my orthopedic doctor's office. Once I was connected to the receptionist, I asked to be transferred to my orthopedic nurse because I had an emergency. The receptionist asked my name and the nature of my call then transferred me. Once I was transferred to the nurse, the recording came on. I left a detailed message with my name and phone number to return my call.

Within an hour, my orthopedic nurse returned my call. I explained to her what was going on with me. She asked me to come in first thing the following morning. She said she was working me in and I would be the first patient my orthopedic would see. I thanked her and hung up.

When we got to the orthopedic office the next morning, I was experiencing so much pain in my left hip, my husband got a wheelchair because he didn't want me walking. For some reason, I could no longer feel the pain in my right hip from the surgery. I don't know if it was because my brain was focused on the left hip and forgot about the right hip, but I no longer felt pain in my right hip. Not long after my husband signed me in, I was called to the back. This time my mother went with us. She sat in the lobby while my husband went to the back with me. My orthopedic doctor came in immediately after we sat down.

"Good morning, dear. What's going on with that left hip of yours?"

"I don't know!" I exclaimed. "I have never experienced pain like this before. It is a different pain from before. It is actually worse!"

"I am going to get an X-ray to see if there has been any change. The radiology technician will be in right away to get you. Don't worry, I am going to do everything I can to take care of you."

"Alright, thank you!"

My orthopedic doctor left the room and the radiology technician came in. He made sure I was the right patient then wheeled me to the radiology room. He helped me onto the cold, flat table and began taking the images. Once he was satisfied with the images, he helped me into the wheelchair and pushed me back to the room where my husband was.

Within minutes after the radiology technician left, my orthopedic doctor came back in.

"I am going to do something that will probably make you want to hit me, but I have to do it."

My husband and I looked at each other and then back at the orthopedic doctor.

"Okay, here we go."

What he did next was unbelievable! He took my left leg and swung it out! I cried out loud in agony!

"I am so sorry! I know it hurts," my doctor said soothingly. "The reason why you are in so much pain and it is different this time is because the bones in your left hip have collapse all the way and they are brittle. They are in tiny pieces. I know I told you and your husband I wanted to wait three to six months to replace the left hip but it's calling for an emergency surgery. I start my vacation the day after tomorrow but I don't want to go on vacation when you need to have surgery. We already had the clearance from your first surgery, so all we need you to do is go ahead and preregister downstairs like you did several weeks ago for your first surgery. I am going to have my nurse send over everything ASAP and by the time you make it downstairs, they will have everything you need to register for surgery.

"Thank you so much," I told him.

"You are more than welcome. I will see you two on April 24."

My husband wheeled me to the lobby where my mother was waiting. The three of us went to pre-admission so I could register for my total left hip replacement surgery. On our way down, my husband explained everything to my mother. She was shocked and surprised I had to have the surgery six weeks after my first surgery. The recovery after a total hip replacement usually takes six months to a year. It is different from case to case.

Once we got to pre-admission, the receptionist noticed I was there no more than six weeks ago for the right hip replacement. She said that after all the years she's worked in pre-admission, she'd never seen a case like mine. She brought up the pre-admission forms for me to sign electronically. Then I was then moved to another area where I had my blood drawn and I provided a urine sample. Last but not least, I saw the last receptionist who specialized in medical billing and coding. We spent several minutes discussing whether my insurance deductible was met yet. When I asked her to look at March 11 when I had my first hip replacement, the days I stayed in the hospital after that and the refund they gave me because I paid up-front before my surgery, the receptionist saw that no money should be taken from me and my deductible was met 100%. She stated anything I would have done in the hospital would be 100% paid by the insurance. She had me sign the forms and pick the type of room I wanted, and we said our goodbyes.

On April 24, 2015, six weeks after my first hip replacement, I was at the hospital hopefully for the last time to get my left hip totally replaced. The process for my second total hip replacement was the same as my first. The only difference this time was that I had different nurses, different certified medical assistants, and different housekeepers assisting me. Of course, it was my orthopedic doctor who performed the surgery for my left hip replacement and his nurse that assisted me.

Once I was in the surgery area getting ready to have my surgery, I remembered the anesthesiologist and what she did before. When she spoke to me and tried to make small talk, I told her with a smile on my face, "I know what you are about to do. You are getting ready to inject that medication into my IV and I am going to be out within seconds and I am not going to see you no more." The orthopedic doctor, his nurse, and the anesthesiologist all laughed at me and said they couldn't get anything past me. By me saying that, this time instead of the anesthesiologist putting the medication in my IV out in the hall, they rolled me into the surgery room. I looked around the big, gigantic room, and saw the surgery tools, all of the gauzes and bandages. I could feel my eyes getting bigger and bigger. My orthopedic doctor asked me if I was ready, and I told him yes. The anesthesiologist injected the medication into my IV and I was out. When I woke up, I was in the recovery room.

My second recovery was a success. I am not 100% pain-free but it is tolerable. Still to this day, I have to use my cane when I leave the house. I have to sit on two pillows and use a plush backrest pillow when I am sitting on the couch. I use the backrest pillow while sitting up in the bed with two pillows under my knees. I have to use two pillows between my legs if I am lying on my side and two pillows under my knees if I am lying on my back. When we go visit family and friends, my husband has to haul the two pillows and my backrest pillows with us. That's the only way I can be comfortable.

Every day after my surgeries was a challenge. I could never predict what my day was going to be like. I have my good days and my bad days. I also have my good nights and my bad nights. I can tell you one thing for sure, I have never gone a day without being in some type of pain. I take medication every day, twice a day.

I also take blood thinners twice a day. The reason for taking the blood thinners is because in early December 2015, I was diagnosed with rare blood clots. It took several appointments to the rheumatologist, over 30 tubes of blood drawn from my veins, and urine collected. Every test the doctor ordered for me came back normal except for the inflammation test. It came back positive because I still have inflammation. The rheumatologist also ordered a few X-rays and MRIs on my lower back, my pelvis and knees because I was complaining about pain in my knees and lower legs. What the rheumatologist explained to me and my husband, we weren't ready nor prepared for. The X-ray showed that the avascular necrosis is now in both of my tibias, or shinbones. (The tibia, or shinbone, is the large bone in the lower front part of the leg, spanning from knee to ankle. Together with the fibula, the tibia connects the ankle to the knee, stabilizing the ankle and providing support to the lower leg muscles.) There was nothing else the rheumatologist could do for me so she referred me to a hematologist.

When I saw the hematologist, she sent me downstairs from her office to the hospital to do labs. She ordered a lot of rare disease tests for me. She thought it could be sickle cell anemia, lupus, or blood clots that were causing the avascular necrosis. Two weeks after I had the blood drawn, I had a follow-up appointment scheduled to see her for my results. Out of the three things she thought I may have that was causing the AVN, one of them was it. My blood results showed I have rare blood clots. The blood clots are causing the rare, silent disease, avascular necrosis.

Diagnostic Tests

Now I am going to share with you all the tests that were performed and what I was tested for by all of the doctors I have seen. This includes images, labs, EKGs, Dopplers, and EMGs. They will be in no specific order and may be repeated more than once.

Blood and urine tests:

Spec Gravity, pH, protein, glucose, Ketone, Bilirubin, Nitrate, Urobilinogen, Leukocyte, Blood, Amphetamine, Barbiturate, Benzodiazepine, Cannabinoid, Cocaine, Opiate, Ur, PCP, Cholesterol, Triglyceride, HDL, LDL, Glucose, Potassium, Urea Nitrogen, Creatinine, GFR, Estimated, GFR, Estim, Afr-Am, TSH, WBC, RBC, Hemoglobin, Hematocrit, MCV, MCH, MCHC, RDW, Platelet, Neutrophil, Lymphocyte, Monocyte, Eosinophil, Basophil, Iron, TIBC, % Iron Sat, Hemoglobin A1c, Est Average Gluc, Free T4, ANA Screen, ANA Titer, ANA Pattern, RA Factor, CO2, Chloride, Potassium, Sodium, Glucose, Urea Nitrogen, Creatinine, Anion Gap, Calcium, GFR, Estimated, GFR, Estim, AFR-Am, Bilirubin, Nitrate, Urobilinogen, Leukocyte, Blood, WBC, RBC, Hemoglobin, Hematocrit, MCV, MCH, MCHC, RDW, Platelet, Neutrophil, Lymphocyte, Monocyte, Eosinophil, Basophil, Neutrophil, Abs, Lymphocyte, Abs, Monocyte, Abs, Eosinophil, Abs, Basophil, Abs, Anti-Cardiolip, IgG, Anti-Cardiolip, IgM, Anti-Cardiolip, IgA, Anti dsDNA, Anti-Smith, ANA Screen, ANA Titer, ANA Pattern, RA Factor, Cholesterol, Triglyceride, HDL, LDL, WBC, LYM, MIO, GRA, LYM%, RBC, HGB, HCT, MCV, MCH, MCHC, RDW, PLT, MPV, Comprehensive Metabolic Panel Glucose, Urea Nitrogen, Egfr Non-AFR, American, Egfr African American, BUN/Creatinine ratio, sodium, potassium, chloride, carbon dioxide, calcium, protein, total, albumin, globulin, albumin/globulin ratio, bilirubin, total, alkaline phosphatase, AST, ALT, TSH, T4, Free, T3, Free, thyroid peroxidase and thyroglobulin antibodies, vitamin B12/folate, ANA Screen IFA, WBC, HGB, HCT, PLT, APTT, INR, PTT, MG, NA, K, CL, CO2, BUN, creatinine, EGFR, glucose, calcium, PHOS, ALKPHOS, BILITOT, BILIDIR, PROT, ALT, AST, sodium, potassium, chloride, CO2, BUN, creatinine, glucose, calcium, EGFR, CBC with platelet, color, UA, Clarity,

UA, specific gravity, UA, pH, UA, protein, UA, glucose, UA, ketones, UA, bilirubin, UA, blood, UA, nitrite, UA, leukocytes, UA, urobilinogen, UA, RBC, UA, WBC, UA, bacteria, UA, squam epithel, UA, WBC, RBC, hemoglobin, hematocrit, MCV, MCH, MCHC, RDW, platelets, MPV, Nrbc, %neutros, %lympphs, %monos, %eos, %baso, #neutros, #lymphs, #monos, #eos, #baso, platelet morphology, atypical lymphs, hypersegmented neutrophils, polychromasia, PT3 PCR, PT, INR, APTT, FIB, RVVT PAT, PTTLA, APC RESISTANCE, TT, FAC VIII, FAC 8 AG, AT3, PROTCFN, PROT C ANTIG, PROT S TOTAL, PROT S FREE, PROT S FUNC, ACA IGG, ACA IGA, ACA IGM, APTABIGG, APTABIGM, APS ABS IGG, APS ABS IGM, APS ABS IGA, BETA-2-IGM, BETA-2-IGG, BETA-2-IGA, HOMOCYSTEINE, HGB A1, HGB A2, HGB S, HGB C, HGB F, HGB SOLUBILITY, HGBINT.

Diagnostic tests:

MRI Lumbar Spine w/o contrast, ECG, chest x-ray, x-ray of bilateral hip (pelvis and lateral hips), EKG, Echocardiogram, right hip x-ray, chest x-ray, MRI pelvis, ECG 12 lead, x-ray hip intraoperative left, EMG

Medications:

Amitriptyline (Elavil), hydrocodone-acetaminophen (Norco), naproxen (Naprosyn), promethazine (Phenergan), prednisone, metoprolol succinate ER, sulfamethoxazole-trimethoprim, levofloxacin (Levaquin), methocarbamol (robaxin), rivaroxaban (Xarelto), solumedrol, amoxicillin-potassium clavulanate

Hospitals/Emergency room visit dates and the reasons for the visit:

March 05, 2005: Leg cramps, bilateral leg cramps
March 06, 2005: Intractable leg pain
November 24, 2013: Left knee pain, hip pain and intractable pain in the left hip
December 20, 2013: Bilateral leg pain

Diagnosis:

Avascular necrosis, right femoral head, total right hip replacement, left femoral head, total left hip replacement, synovium with chronic inflammation, rare blood clots.

Epilogue

I am now living my life second by second, minute by minute, hour by hour, day by day and night by night. I never know what my morning, day or night will be like. Sometimes it surprises me.

I was told by all of my doctors not to drink alcohol. I have never been a big alcohol drinker anyway. I used to only drink occasionally, but since my doctors told me to never drink alcohol again because it could kill me, I have not had an alcohol drink since July 4, 2013. I take all of my medications as directed. I do what my doctors instruct me to do.

I had both of my hips totally replaced at the age of 39. I am now a stay-at-home wife and mother with a seven-year-old Bichon named Trixter.

I write short stories every chance I get. I set a goal to have each short story finished because if I didn't, I would prolong doing it and that to me is like giving up. Just because I am no longer physically able to go out and work like I used to, drive a car like I used to, walk around grocery stores like I used to, walk around department stores or even a mall like I used to, I still on a daily basis try to keep myself occupied mentally at all times because being limited to what I can and can't do is something I am still trying to get used to.

I used to be an energetic person that never stopped going until I got in my bed at night. But now, sometimes I am in bed all day. But guess what, I push myself to write anyway. I am not going to let rare blood clots and avascular necrosis get the best of me. I am already ahead of it!

I wanted to go back to school and get my license to practice psychiatry before I got sick. Well, that didn't happen.

I tried everything to keep myself busy. Pinterest was my best friend. You see, Pinterest has step-by-step directions on how to do anything you want to do. For my 41st birthday, our oldest son bought me a sewing machine, and our youngest son bought some accessories for the sewing machine. I bought material from different stores because I wanted to make quilts, rugs, shower curtains, and curtains but instead I made my niece a lot of barrettes, I made pinecone wreaths, and I painted pinecones. I got bored with those things fast so I pulled out my nook and started reading book after book after book.

One day a light bulb went off in my head. I told my husband, our sons, my mom, my sisters, my nieces, my best friend and my son's girlfriend I was going to write a book. I knew in their minds they were thinking I wasn't just talking because they knew me and they knew if I said I was going to do something, I was going to do it.

Look at me now! I HAVE MY FAMILY AND CLOSEST FRIENDS. THAT IS MY MOTIVATION AND MY INSPIRATION! BACK OFF, RARE BLOOD CLOTS AND AVASCULAR NECROSIS (AVN), I AM WINNING!

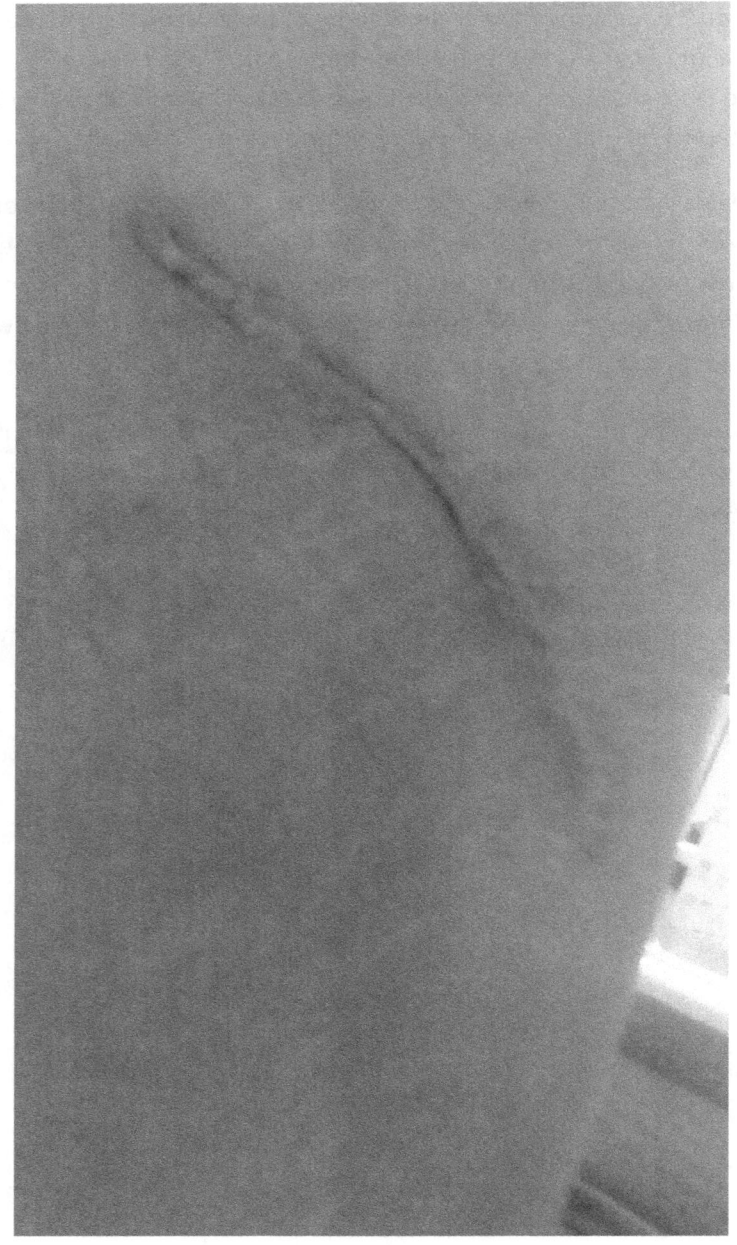

This is the surgery site of my first total hip replacement (right hip).

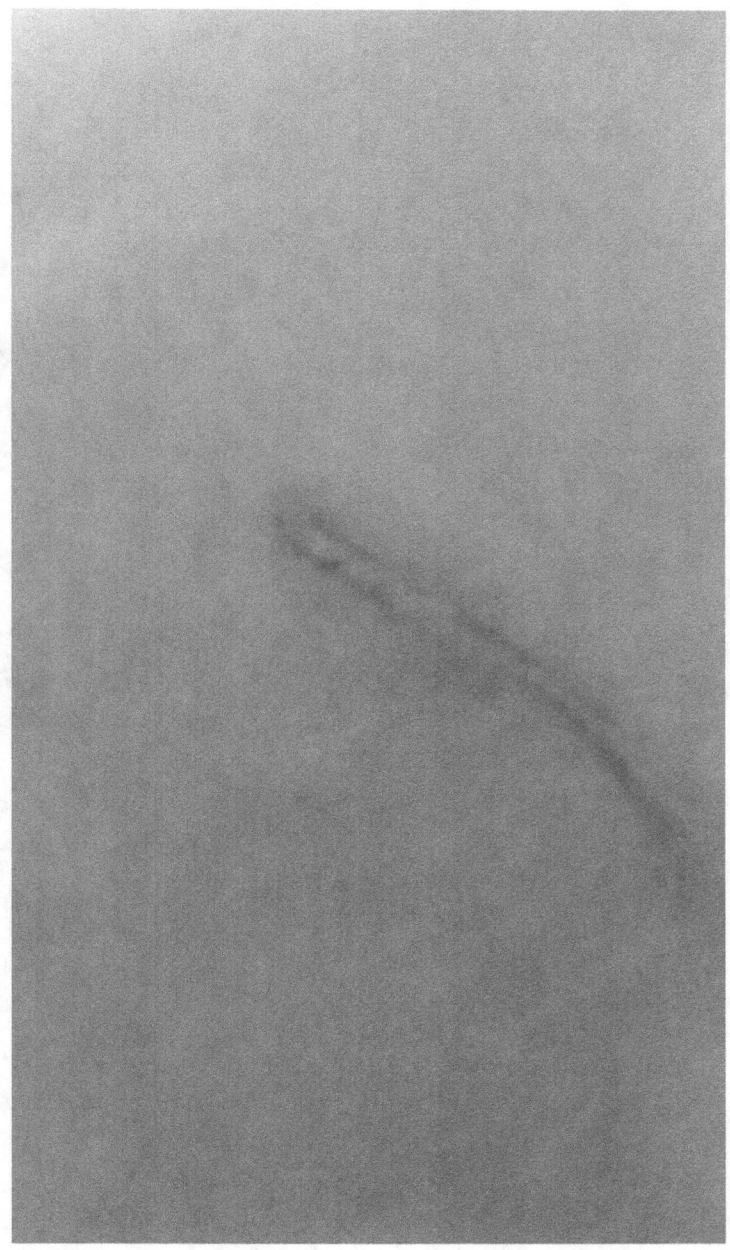

This is the surgery site of my second total hip replacement (left hip).

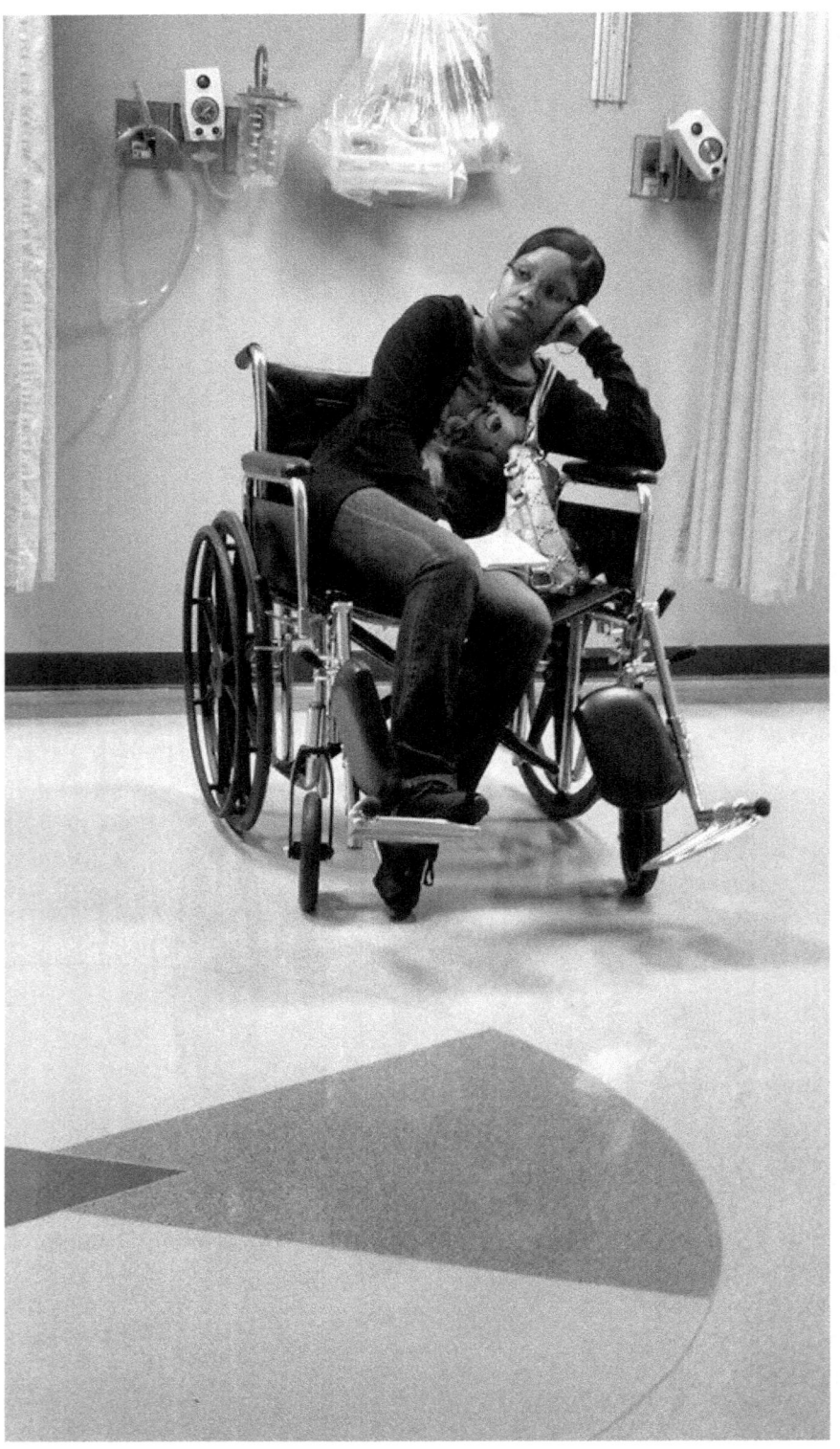

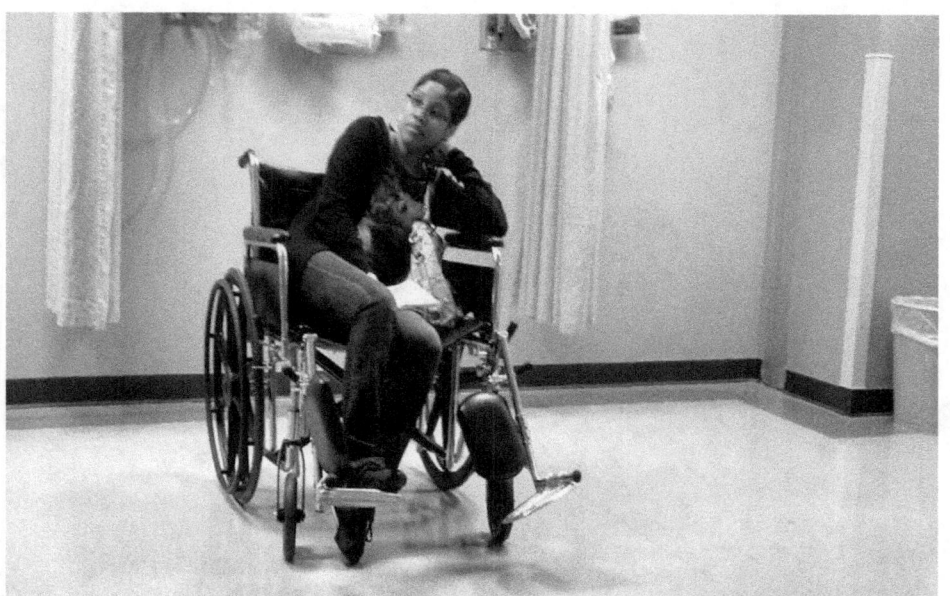

Patiently waiting in the Emergency Room area for my scans.

Still waiting for my scans in the Emergency Room waiting area.

WYKETHA K PARKMAN

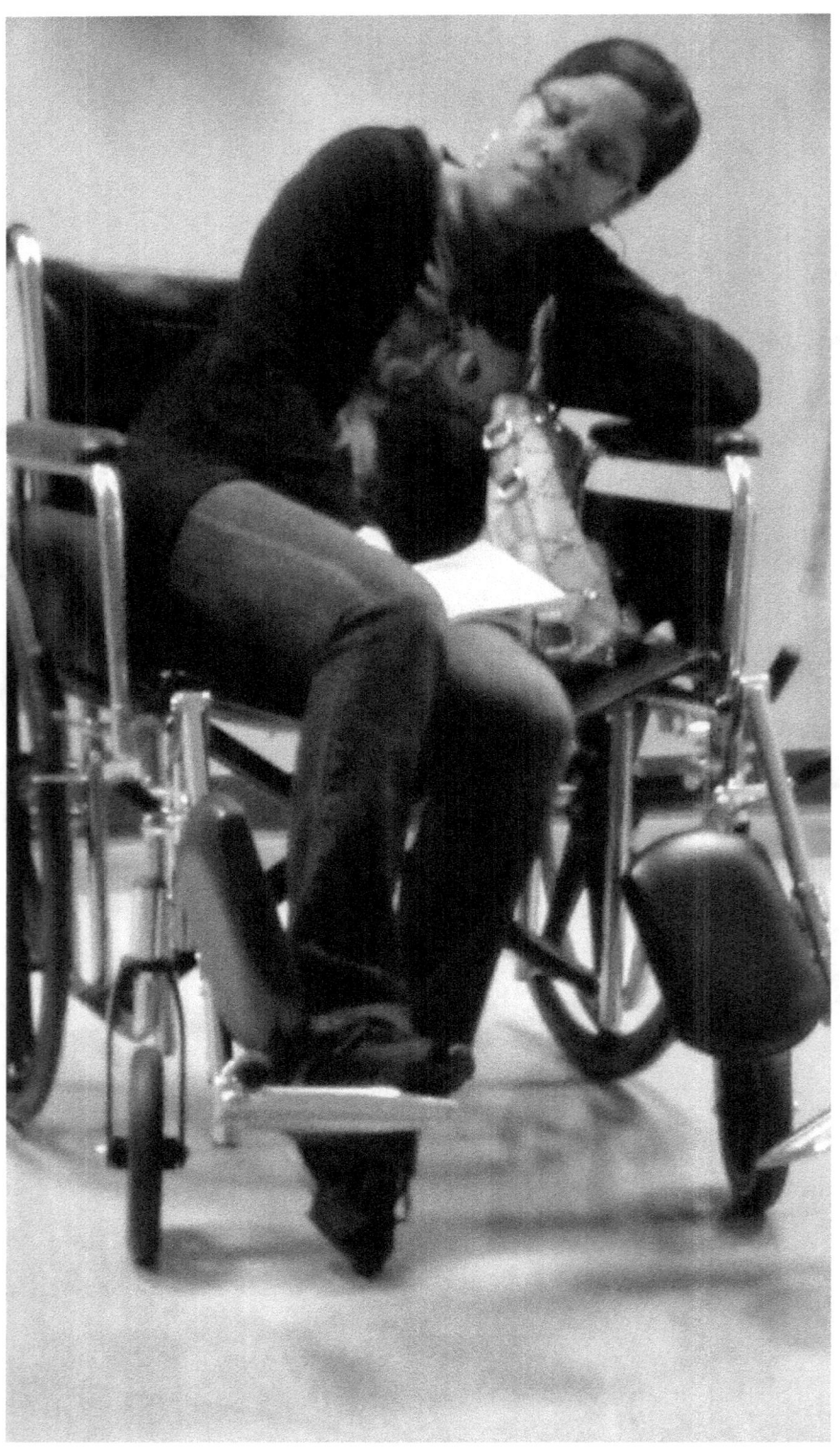

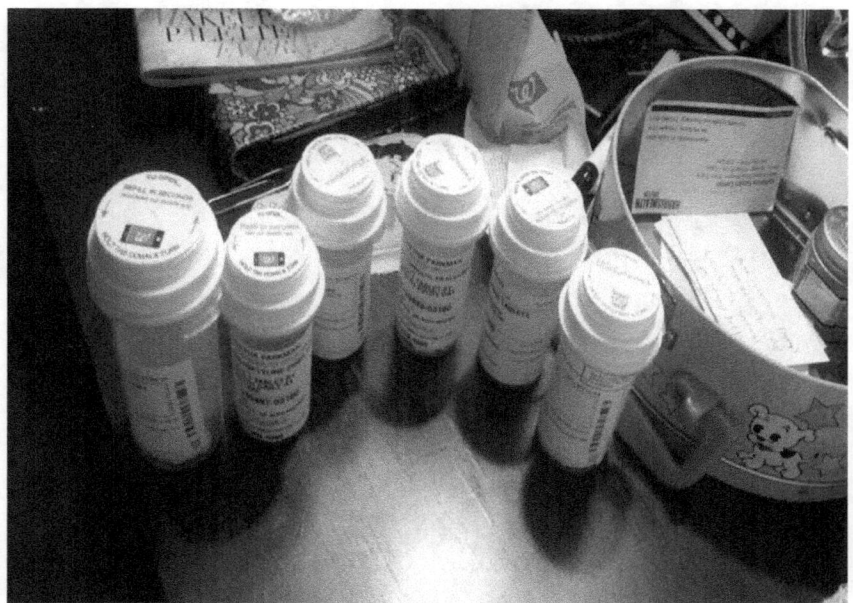

During this time, the pain was excruciating.

Some of the medication I was on prior to being diagnosed.

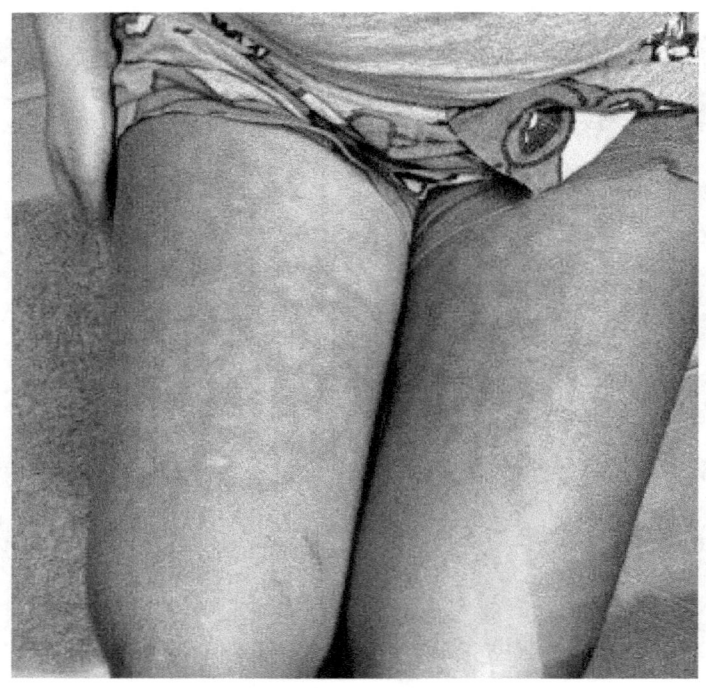

In this image, you can see the purple, speckled, zigzag lines and swelling on both of my legs.

About the author

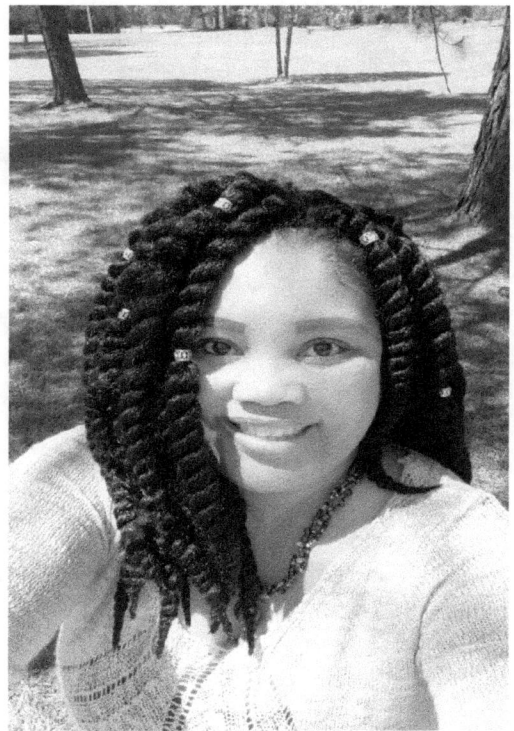

After working thirteen years in the medical field, I am now a stay-at-home wife with two adult sons and a five year old Bischon (dog) name Trixter, who I adore and love dearly, who enjoy spending all of my spare time on reading and writing.

You can find all of my books at any of the online sites below:

www.amazon.com/author/wykethaparkman

www.goodreads.com/authorwkp

www.facebook.com/authorwkp

Books A Million

Barnes and Noble

Nook

Kindle

You can follow me:

www.amazon.com/author/wykethaparkman

www.goodreads.com/authorwkp

https://fb.me/authorWykethaParkman

@authorwkp

Please don't forget to rate and write a review. You can do so by clicking below.

www.amazon.com/author/wykethaparkman

I started a petition to acknowledge Avascular Necrosis for it's disabling state. Please help me getting this approve by the White House by clicking on the link below. All is needed is your first and last name, email address and zip code. You can share the petition via email and text. Let's make this happen.

Thank you in advance.

https://sign.moveon.org/petitions/awareness-for-the-disease

Avascular Necrosis 8.5 xx 11 Journal available for purchase on Amazon.

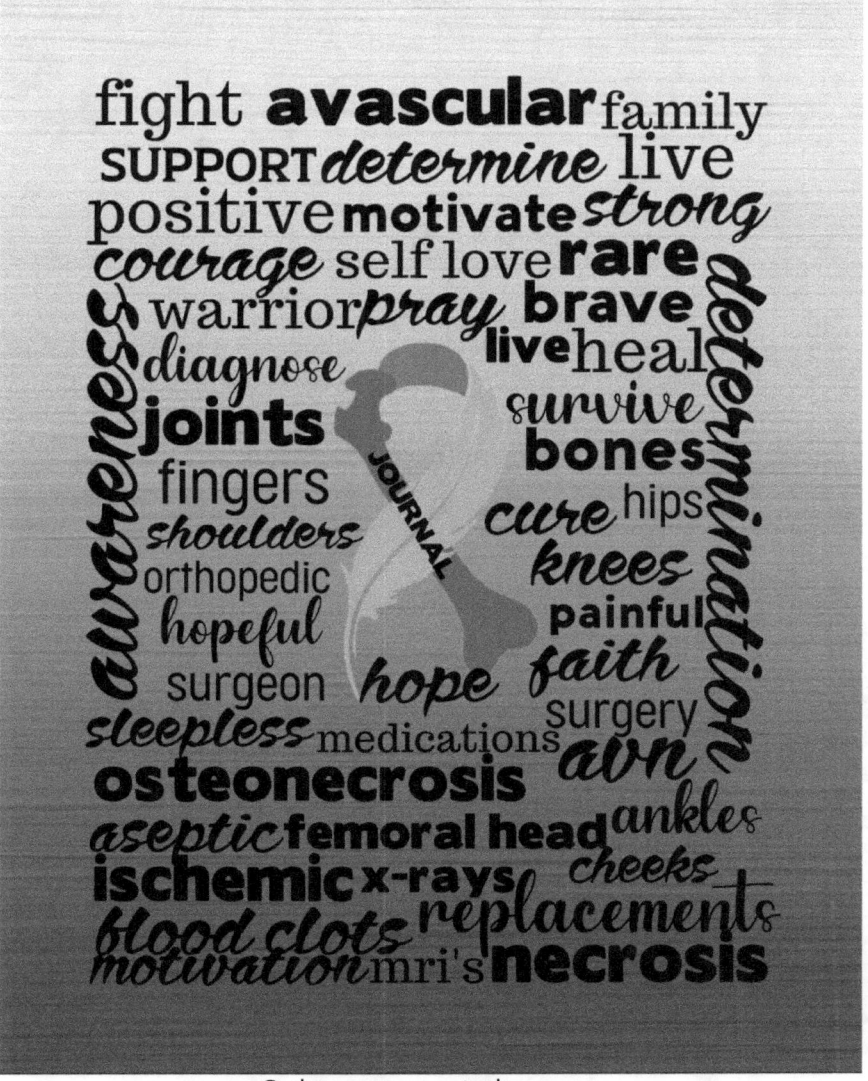

Order your copy today.